YOGA FOR PREGNANT WOMEN:

"Blossoming Serenity: Nurturing Yoga Practices for Every Trimester"

Dr. Vera J. Reynolds

Copyright

Contents

INTRODUCTION

Embarking on the magical adventure of pregnancy is a time of tremendous change, both for the body and the spirit. As you nourish a new life inside you, the link between mind, body, and soul becomes more nuanced and precious than ever before. In the middle of this incredible chapter, there exists a gentle companion that can accompany you through the ebbs and flows of your journey: yoga. Welcome to the realm of "Yoga for Pregnant Women," where the ancient knowledge of yoga delicately intertwines with the wonder of life.

Picture yourself enclosed in a calm place, a refuge that celebrates the trip you are making. Here, yoga becomes more than simply a physical practice—it becomes a caring refuge where you enjoy the energy of each breath, the power in your evolving shape, and the whispers of intuition that echo from inside. "Yoga for Pregnant Women" is more than a practice—embracing self-love, a celebration of the deep connection between your body and the child it cradles.

Within the pages of this book, you'll unearth a harmonic symphony of postures, breathwork, and mindfulness that cater to your ever-evolving requirements. From calming stretches that ease pregnancy aches to breathing methods that welcome tranquillity, each chapter is a thoughtfully written invitation to experience the symbiotic dance between motherhood and yoga. As you travel through the trimesters, you'll learn how yoga adapts, accepting your body's changes while fostering your spirit's development.

Let this handbook be your trusty companion—a source of peace, strength, and self-discovery. As you enter the realm of "Yoga for

Pregnant Women," may you discover physical refreshment and the empowerment that comes from recognizing the intrinsic knowledge of your body. With each exercise, you'll establish a stronger connection to your baby, your breath, and the everlasting rhythm of life itself. Welcome to a transforming journey that harmonizes the art of yoga with the wonder of motherhood—where each position becomes a prayer and each breath a song of love.

CHAPTER ONE

Benefits of Yoga for Pregnant Women

Following are some of the primary advantages of practising yoga for pregnant women:

1. Physical Well-being:

- **Improved Flexibility:** Yoga helps to maintain and enhance flexibility in muscles and joints, which may be particularly useful during pregnancy when the body experiences changes.
- **Enhanced Strength:** Yoga postures concentrate on strengthening strength, which may assist in bearing the additional weight of pregnancy and preparing the body for delivery.
- **Better Posture:** Practicing yoga may help pregnant women maintain excellent posture, minimizing tension on the back and nook.

2. Stress Reduction:

- **Relaxation methods:** Yoga combines deep Breathing, meditation, and relaxation methods that may help manage stress and anxiety, generating a feeling of peace.
- **Cortisol Regulation:** Yoga may help manage cortisol levels, the stress hormone, leading to a more serene state of mind.

3. Pain Relief:

- **Back Pain Alleviation:** Yoga helps ease back pain and stiffness typically encountered during pregnancy by gently stretching and strengthening the back muscles.
- **Sciatica Management:** Certain yoga positions may relieve sciatic nerve discomfort, a frequent condition in pregnancy.

4. Bonding with the Baby:

- **Conscious Connection:** Prenatal yoga allows pregnant moms to build a conscious connection with their unborn baby, promoting a feeling of closeness and love.

5. Labor Preparation:

- **Breathing Techniques:** Yoga emphasizes deep and regulated Breathing, which may be good during labour and delivery to manage discomfort and remain calm.
- **Pelvic Floor Awareness:** Certain postures and movements in prenatal yoga help promote awareness and strength of the pelvic floor muscles, assisting in labour and postpartum healing.

6. Improved Circulation:

- **Blood Flow Enhancement:** Yoga positions enhance healthy blood circulation, minimizing the risk of swelling and varicose veins frequently linked with pregnancy.

7. Digestive Health:

- **Relief from Digestive Issues:** Gentle yoga positions and twists may assist with digestion, helping to reduce typical pregnancy-related digestive discomforts.

8. Positive Mindset:

- **Confidence increase:** Practicing yoga during pregnancy may increase a woman's self-confidence and body image as she adjusts to her changing body.

9. Better Sleep:

- **Sleep Quality Improvement:** Relaxation practices in yoga may enhance sleep quality, addressing the sleep disruptions that some pregnant women suffer.

10. Social Support:

- **Community:** Joining prenatal yoga sessions allows pregnant women to interact with others going through a similar journey, bringing emotional support and camaraderie.

11. Postpartum Recovery:

- **Faster Recovery:** Maintaining a yoga practice throughout pregnancy might lead to a speedier postpartum recovery, assisting in recovering strength and flexibility.

Safety Precautions and Guidelines

Here are some safety considerations and tips to follow while practising yoga as a pregnant woman:

1. **Visit Your Healthcare Provider:** Before beginning any fitness regimen, including yoga, visit your healthcare provider to confirm that it's safe for you and your baby, particularly if you have any medical concerns or difficulties.

2. **Choose Prenatal Yoga sessions:** Opt for sessions mainly developed for pregnant women or guided by teachers with expertise in prenatal yoga. They will be acquainted with positions that are safe and healthy during pregnancy.

3. **Listen to Your Body:**
- Pay special attention to how your body feels throughout each posture.
- If anything seems unpleasant, stop immediately.
- Never push yourself to the point of discomfort or strain.

4. **Modify positions:** Many conventional yoga positions may be adjusted to fit your changing physique. Use props like blocks, bolsters, and straps to assist your practice and make classes more accessible.

5. **Avoid Overstretching:** The hormone relaxin is produced during pregnancy, which might make your joints more flexible. Be careful not to overstretch since this might lead to damage.

6. **Avoid Deep Twists and Backbends:** Deep twists and backbends should be undertaken with care during pregnancy. These positions might squeeze the abdomen and strain the ligaments.

7. **No Supine Positions After the First Trimester:** After the first trimester, avoid positions that involve laying flat on your back for a lengthy time since this might obstruct blood flow to the uterus.

8. **Pelvic Floor Awareness:** Focus on activating and strengthening your pelvic floor muscles. This may be good for both labour and postpartum rehabilitation.

9. **Breathing:** Incorporate deep and regulated breathing methods. Practice calm, deliberate Breathing to help control stress and remain relaxed.

10. **Hydration and Nutrition:** Stay hydrated before, during, and after your yoga session. Eat a small snack if required to maintain your energy levels.

11. **Avoid Inversions:** Inversions like headstands and shoulder stands should typically be avoided during pregnancy because of the greater danger of falling and the strain they impose on the abdomen.

12. **Stay Cool:** Avoid practising in warm environments since your body temperature increases during pregnancy. Overheating may be risky for both you and your baby.

13. **Gear:** Wear comfortable, breathable gear that allows you a complete range of motion. Maternity-specific yoga clothing may give additional support for your developing belly.

14. **Remain Hydrated:** Drink water before, during, and after your practice to stay hydrated.

15. **Relax:** Don't hesitate to pause and relax whenever you need to. Your body works hard to sustain your pregnancy, so heed its signs.

Remember that every pregnancy is unique, so what works for one woman may not be acceptable for another. It's always advisable to err on the side of caution and emphasize safety for you and your kid. If you're confused about any part of your yoga practice during pregnancy, visit your healthcare practitioner or a qualified prenatal yoga teacher.

CHAPTER TWO

Preparing Mind and Body for Prenatal Yoga

Mental and Emotional Preparation

Mental and emotional preparation are crucial components of pregnancy, and practising yoga may be a beneficial tool to assist your well-being during this transforming period. Here are some advice and practices for mental and emotional preparation with yoga:

1. **Mindfulness Meditation:** Incorporate mindfulness meditation into your practice. This practice helps you remain present, decrease stress, and establish a stronger connection with your body and baby.

2. **Breathing methods:** Learn and practice several breathing methods, such as deep belly breathing, ujjayi breath, and alternate nostril breathing. These approaches may quiet your mind, decrease worry, and give relaxation.

3. **Visualization:** Use visualization methods to prepare for labour and delivery psychologically. Visualize a pleasant birth experience, envisioning yourself strong and confident throughout the procedure.

4. **Positive Affirmations:** Create and repeat positive affirmations about pregnancy, delivery, and parenthood. These affirmations enhance your confidence and encourage a good outlook.

5. **Journaling:** Keep a pregnant diary to capture your emotions, experiences, and thoughts. Writing may be therapeutic and help you process your feelings.

6. **Restorative Yoga:** Practice restorative yoga to relax your body and mind thoroughly. These soft postures are ideal for alleviating stress and enhancing mental well-being.

7. **Chanting & Mantras:** Incorporate chanting or repeating mantras that connect with you. The repetition of sounds or phrases may have a relaxing effect and enhance attention.

8. **Yoga Nidra:** Try yoga nidra, also known as yogic slumber. This guided meditation technique generates profound relaxation and may be especially beneficial for alleviating anxiety.

9. **Welcome Changes:** Use yoga to promote self-acceptance and welcome changes in your body. Gentle stretches and postures help you feel more comfortable with your shifting body.

10. **Self-Care Rituals:** Create self-care rituals incorporating yoga, such as morning or evening routines. These routines create a feeling of consistency and help you retain a good mindset.

11. **Community Connection:** Join prenatal yoga classes or support groups to connect with other pregnant moms. Sharing experiences and hardships may build a feeling of kinship and support.

12. **Letting Go:** Use yoga to master the skill of letting go. Release any concerns or anxiety regarding pregnancy, delivery, and parenthood via breathwork and movement.

13. **Gratitude Practice:** Cultivate a gratitude practice. Focus on the good parts of your pregnancy experience and show gratitude for the changes.

14. **Mindful Movement:** Approach your yoga practice as a moving meditation. Pay special attention to each movement, building a stronger mind-body connection.

15. **Kind Self-Compassion:** Be kind to oneself. Pregnancy may bring a multitude of feelings. Allow yourself to feel these emotions without judgment.

Remember that pregnancy is a period of significant transition, both physically and mentally. Your mental and emotional well-being are equally as vital as your physical health. Incorporating yoga practices into your regimen may equip you with skills to negotiate the dynamic elements of pregnancy with more comfort and happiness. If you feel that your emotional issues become overwhelming, consider obtaining help from a mental health specialist specializing in perinatal care.

Physical Preparations and Modifications

Physical preparation and adaptations in yoga during pregnancy are vital to protect your and your baby's safety and comfort. Here are some recommendations and tweaks for tailoring your yoga practice to your changing body:

1. **Warm-Up:** Begin each session with a mild introduction to prepare your body for activity. Focus on moderate stretches and deep Breathing.

2. **Use Props:** Utilize props such as blocks, bolsters, and straps to assist your practice. Braces help you maintain appropriate alignment and avoid overstretching.

3. **Focus on Stability:** Emphasize positions that promote stability and balance. Poses like Warrior II, Tree Pose, and Modified Triangle Pose might be helpful.

4. **Avoid Deep Twists:** Avoid deep twisting positions, particularly in the stomach region. Gentle twists that don't squeeze the tummy are safer.

5. **Modify Forward Folds:** Modify forward folding postures by keeping your legs more expansive and bending your knees. This avoids tension in your lower back and accommodates your increasing tummy.

6. **Pelvic Floor Awareness:** Incorporate pelvic floor awareness and engagement activities to support the pelvic area and prepare for labour.

7. **Avoid Deep Backbends:** Avoid deep backbends that compress the abdomen. Opt for softer backbends like Cat-Cow or supported Bridge Pose.

8. **Supine positions:** After the first trimester, avoid situations that involve resting flat on your back for lengthy durations. Use props to lift your upper body.

9. **Inversions:** Avoid inversions like headstands and shoulder stands since they may place too much strain on the abdomen and impair blood flow.

10. **Squatting positions:** Incorporate squatting positions like Goddess Pose or supported Malasana to prepare for birth and expand the hips.

11. **Use Chairs:** Chairs may support positions like squats and forward folds. They assist you in retaining balance and equilibrium.

12. **Practice Wall Postures:** Wall postures like Wall Plank and Wall Warrior II may give support and stability while keeping perfect alignment.

13. **Gentle Flow:** Opt for a gentle flow practice emphasizing smooth transitions between postures rather than aggressive movements.

14. **Restorative positions:** Integrate beneficial classes like Savasana (Corpse Pose) with bolsters and blankets to soothe your body and mind.

15. **Listen to Your Body:** Pay heed to your body's messages. If a position is unpleasant or painful, alter or skip it.

16. **Keep Hydrated:** Keep water available and keep hydrated during your practice.

17. **Breathe Awareness:** Focus on your breath throughout each position. Deep, steady Breathing may help you remain calm and concentrated.

18. **Regular pauses:** Take pauses as required, particularly if you feel exhausted. Don't push yourself too much.

19. **Cool Down:** Finish each practice with a cooling-down routine that involves mild stretches and relaxation.

20. **Regular Check-ins:** As your pregnancy advances, your requirements may alter. Regularly examine how you feel and make modifications appropriately.

Pregnancy is a unique adventure, and every woman's experience is distinct. It's crucial to emphasize your comfort and safety at all times. If you need clarification about changes or have particular concerns, try practising under the direction of a professional prenatal yoga teacher who can give tailored instruction.

CHAPTER THREE

Breathing Techniques for Relaxation and Stress Relief

Breathing exercises, or pranayama, may be beneficial for relaxation and stress alleviation during pregnancy. Here are several breathing exercises that you may use to help relax your mind, decrease worry, and create a feeling of well-being:

Deep Belly Breathing (Diaphragmatic Breathing)

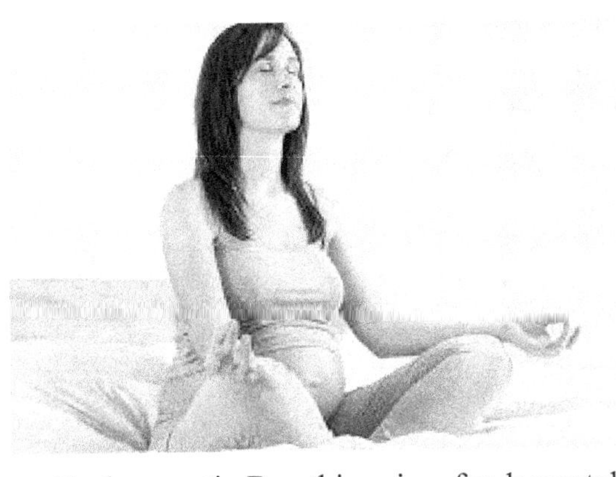

Deep belly breathing, or diaphragmatic Breathing, is a fundamental breathing technique that promotes relaxation, decreases stress, and boosts general well-being. It's a simple but effective exercise that may be especially useful during pregnancy. Here's how to conduct deep belly breathing:

1. **Find a Comfortable posture:** Sit or lay down in a comfortable posture. If lying down, you may position a cushion or pillow beneath your head and legs.

2. **Relax Your Body:** Close your eyes if you're comfortable, and take a minute to relax your body. Let go of any tightness in your muscles.

3. **Place Your Hands:** Rest one hand on your chest and the other on your abdomen, right below your ribs.

4. **Breathe slowly:** Take a slow and gentle breath through your nose. Focus on letting your breath go deep into your abdomen rather than elevating your chest.

5. **Feel the Belly Rise:** Your belly expands and rises as you inhale. It would help if you observed your hand on your tummy rising higher while the hand on your chest stays relatively static.

6. **Exhale Gradually:** Slowly exhale through your nose. Feel your tummy fall and clench as you release the breath.

7. **Continue the Pattern:** Continue breathing deeply through your nose, allowing your belly to rise and exhaling slowly, feeling your stomach fall.

8. **Maintain a Smooth Rhythm:** Focus on maintaining a smooth and equal rhythm of breath. Inhale and exhale at a comfortable rate.

9. **Be Present:** As you practice, strive to be present and involved in the sensations of your breath. Let go of any distracting notions.

10. **Practice time:** Start with a few minutes of deep belly breathing and progressively extend the time as you feel more comfortable.

Benefits:

- Deep belly breathing induces relaxation by activating the parasympathetic nervous system, sometimes called the "rest and digest" mode.
- It helps alleviate stress, anxiety, and tension, which may be helpful during pregnancy.
- This strategy promotes oxygen intake, which supports your and your kid's health.
- Deep belly breathing may strengthen your mind-body connection and awareness.

It's a primary method that can be done anywhere and anytime.

Incorporate deep belly breathing into your everyday routine, particularly when you feel anxious, overwhelmed, or need relaxation. Regular practice may have a favourable influence on your entire feeling of well-being throughout pregnancy.

Ujjayi Breath (Victorious Breath)

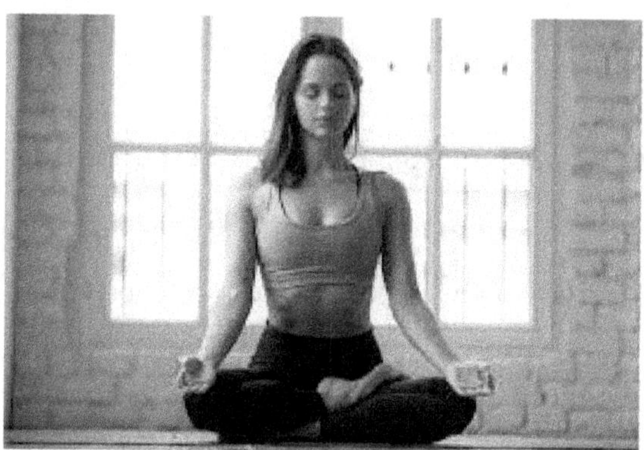

Ujjayi breath, frequently referred to as "Victorious Breath," is a pranayama method often utilized in yoga. It includes a slight tightening of the throat to make a gentle, audible sound during inhale and exhale. This breath method may help quiet the mind, regulate the breath, and generate a sensation of relaxation and concentration. Here's how to practice Ujjayi breath:

Steps:

1. **Find a Comfortable Seat:** Sit in a comfortable cross-legged posture or on a chair with your spine erect. You may also practice Ujjayi breath while lying down.

2. **Relax and Close Your Eyes:** Close your eyes lightly if you're comfortable, and take a minute to relax your face muscles and shoulders.

3. **Inhale Through Your Nose:** Start by taking a calm, deep breath in through your nose. As you inhale, restrict the back of

your throat slightly. It's comparable to the experience of fogging up a mirror with your breath.

4. **Create the Sound:** As you inhale, produce a quiet "ha" sound in your throat. This sound should be delicate and soothing, like the sound of the ocean waves or a calm snoring.

5. **Exhale Through Your Nose:** Exhale gently through your nose while keeping the same slight constriction of your throat. Again, you should hear the gentle "ha" sound.

6. **Maintain a Steady Rhythm:** Continue this cycle of Breathing and exhaling through your nose, generating the ocean-like sound in your throat. The sound should be constant and rhythmic.

7. **Regulate the Breath:** Focus on managing the duration of your inhales and exhales. Make them equal in length and comfortable for you. You may start with a count of four for both inhalation and exhalation.

8. **Keep attentive:** As you practice, stay alert to the feeling of the breath, the sound you're generating, and the relaxing impact it has on your mind.

Benefits:

- Ujjayi breath helps to regulate and slow down the breath, which may have a soothing impact on the nervous system.
- The audible sound of Ujjayi breath may serve as a focus point for your meditation practice, helping to anchor your attention.

- This breath method increases awareness, helping you remain present and focused throughout your yoga practice.
- Ujjayi breath facilitates more profound lung expansion, enhancing oxygen intake and a calm sensation.
- It may be especially beneficial in reducing stress, anxiety, and restlessness.

Note: *While Ujjayi breath is typically safe for most people, practising it without straining your throat is crucial. If you encounter any pain or dizziness, return to your usual breath. Check with your healthcare physician before practising Ujjayi breath if you have any respiratory ailments or concerns.*

Incorporate Ujjayi breath into your yoga practice, particularly during asana (posture) practice or meditation. With repeated practice, you'll get more comfortable with the method and feel its relaxing advantages.

Box Breathing (Square Breathing)

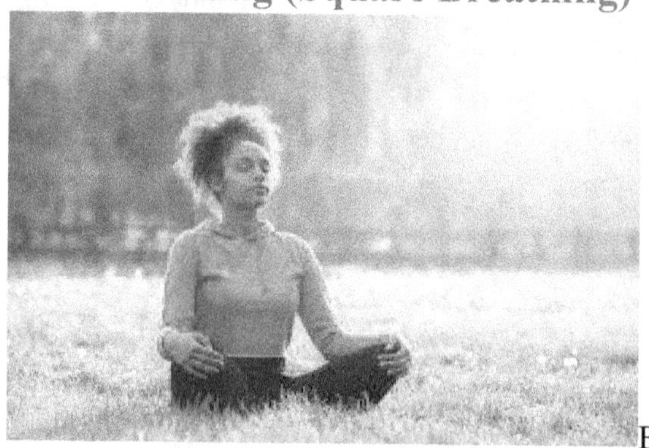

Box breathing, also known as square Breathing, is a simple and effective respiratory control method that may be safely done throughout pregnancy to induce relaxation, decrease stress, and manage anxiety. Here's how you can alter box breathing during pregnancy:

1. **Find a Comfortable Position:** Sit in a comfortable chair or on the floor with your back straight. You can also lie down on your side if that's more comfortable.

2. **Relax Your Shoulders:** Allow your shoulders to relax and softly shut your eyes if you're comfortable doing so.

3. **Inhale Slowly:** Inhale through your nose slowly and steadily for a count of four. As you inhale, picture filling your gut with air, allowing it to expand.

4. **Hold Your Breath:** After inhaling, hold your breath for a count of four. During this breath holding, keep a comfortable and stable posture.

5. **Exhale Gradually:** Exhale through your nose for a count of four, allowing your tummy to contract as you release the breath gently.

6. **Wait before Inhaling:** After exhaling, wait for a count of four before inhaling again. This time of silence builds the "box" shape of the breath rhythm.

7. **Repeat the Cycle:** Continue this cycle of Breathing for four counts, holding for four counts, exhaling for four counts, and

stopping for four counts. You may modify the count to a pleasant rhythm if desired.

Benefits:

- Box breathing may assist in soothing the neurological system and lowering tension and anxiety.
- It's a primary and accessible method that can be done anywhere and anytime.
- This approach fosters attention and presence, helping you remain connected to the present moment.
- Box breathing gives your breath a regular and rhythmic pattern, assisting in relaxation and attention.

Safety Precautions:

- Box breathing is typically safe for pregnant women. However, if you suffer any dizziness, shortness of breath, or pain, quit the exercise and return to your usual Breathing.
- Practice box breathing in a well-ventilated place to ensure you're obtaining adequate oxygen.

Tips:

- Practice box breathing for a few minutes or longer, depending on your comfort level.
- If you find it tough to hold your breath for four counts, you may cut the period to two or three counts.
- Box breathing may be a great technique to help you handle pregnancy's physical and mental changes.

Alternate Nostril Breathing (Nadi Shodhana)

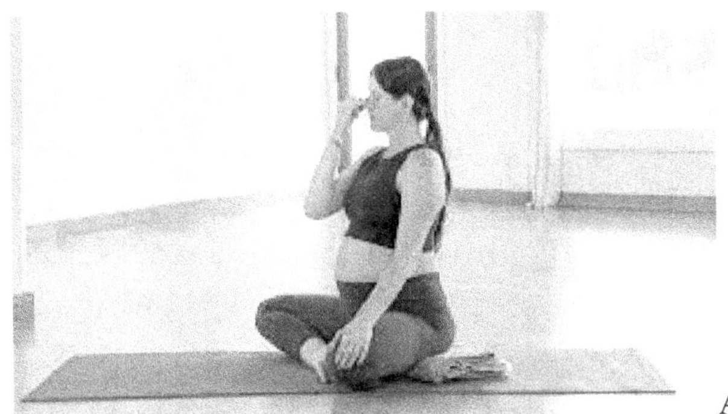

Alternate Nostril Breathing, or Nadi Shodhana or Anulom Vilom, is a balanced and relaxing pranayama method that may be done throughout pregnancy to increase relaxation, decrease tension, and enhance breath awareness. However, there are a few adaptations and concerns to bear in mind to guarantee the safety and comfort of both you and your baby:

Steps:

1. **Find a Comfortable Seat:** Sit comfortably with your back straight. You may sit cross-legged on the floor or a chair. Ensure your spine is aligned.

2. **Relax Your Shoulders:** Allow your shoulders to relax and softly shut your eyes if you're comfortable doing so.

3. **Hand Position:** Rest your left hand on your left knee with your palm facing up. Use your right thumb to seal your right nostril gently.

4. **Inhale Through Your Left Nostril:** Begin breathing deeply and gently through your left nostril. Close your right nostril with your right thumb while you do this.

5. **Switch Nostrils:** After breathing, release your right nostril and use your right ring finger to seal your left nostril gently.

6. **Exhale via Your Right Nostril:** Exhale gently and thoroughly via your right nostril. Keep your left nostril closed while you exhale.

7. **Inhale Through Your Right Nostril:** Inhale deeply through your right nostril while keeping your left nostril closed.

8. **Switch Nostrils Again:** Release your left nostril and softly seal your right nostril with your right thumb.

9. **Exhale via Your Left Nostril:** Exhale gently and thoroughly via your left nostril.

10. **Repeat the Cycle:** Continue this cycle of Breathing through one nostril, switching, and exhaling through the other nose. Start and end with an inhale via your left nostril.

Modifications and Considerations:

1. **Gentle Breathing:** Practice alternate nostril breathing softly and without force during pregnancy. The breath should flow easily and naturally.

2. **Avoid Breath Retention:** While specific variants of Nadi Shodhana require breath retention, it's better to avoid holding your breath for lengthy durations during pregnancy.

3. **Avoid Strain:** If you feel discomfort, strain, or dizziness, quit the practice and return to regular Breathing.

4. **Practice Moderately:** You may practice alternate nostril breathing for a few minutes daily or as part of your pranayama practice.

Benefits:

- Alternate Nostril Breathing helps balance the energy pathways in the body, giving a sensation of serenity and stability.
- It helps promote breath awareness and mindfulness, which can be especially effective during pregnancy.
- This approach aids relaxation, decreases tension, and facilitates a concentrated and centred state of mind.

As with any pranayama practice during pregnancy, it's vital to check your healthcare professional before beginning or maintaining a new breathing method. If you have any worries, medical issues, or pain, it's encouraged to practice under the instruction of a professional prenatal yoga instructor or a skilled pranayama teacher.

4-7-8 Breathing

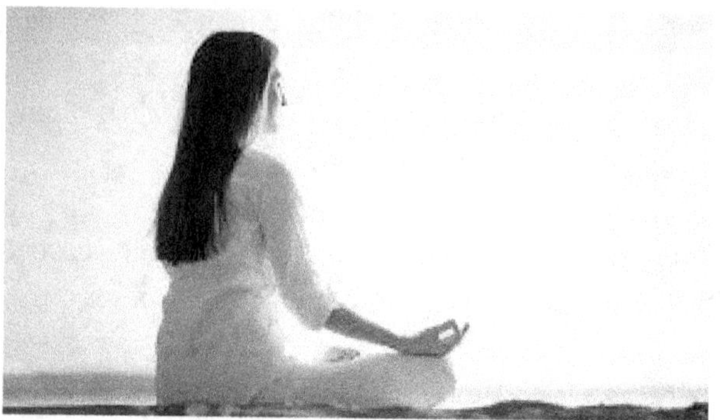

The 4-7-8 breathing method, commonly known as "relaxing breath," may be a beneficial relaxation exercise during pregnancy when used attentively and gently. However, like any breathing technique during pregnancy, it's crucial to make adaptations to fit your specific requirements. Here's how you may alter the 4-7-8 breathing method during pregnancy:

Steps:

1. **Find a Comfortable posture:** Sit or lay down in a comfortable posture. You may sit cross-legged, on a chair, or lay on your side with a cushion for support.

2. **Relax Your Shoulders:** Allow your shoulders to relax and softly shut your eyes if you're comfortable doing so.

3. **Inhale for Four Counts:** Inhale gently through your nose for a count of four. Focus on filling your lungs slowly and naturally.

4. **Hold for Comfort:** Hold your breath for a comfortable count. During pregnancy, you may alter the count to fit what seems comfortable. It can be a maximum of seven counts if that seems too lengthy.

5. **Exhale for Eight Counts:** Exhale slowly and thoroughly via your mouth or nose for a count of eight. Feel your body release tension with each inhalation.

6. **Repeat the Cycle:** Continue this cycle of inhaling for a count of four, holding for a count that feels comfortable, and exhaling for a count of eight.

Modifications and Considerations:

1. **Adapt the numbers:** If the 4-7-8 ratio doesn't seem right for you throughout pregnancy, you may change the numbers. For example, you may drill 3-5-6 or 4-6-8. The objective is to generate a peaceful rhythm that doesn't induce pain.

2. **Comfortable Breath Retention:** If breath retention seems unpleasant, concentrate on deep inhalations and exhalations without holding your breath.

Benefits:

- The 4-7-8 breathing method may assist in quieting the nervous system and induce relaxation.
- It stimulates slower, deeper Breathing, which may be suitable for lowering tension and anxiety.
- This technique may be readily implemented into your everyday routine to produce moments of quiet and tranquillity.

- If you suffer any dizziness, shortness of breath, or discomfort, quit the exercise and return to your usual Breathing.
- If you have any medical ailments or concerns, visit your healthcare practitioner before trying new breathing methods during pregnancy.

Pregnancy is a unique adventure; what works for one person may not work for another. Listen to your body and practice inside your comfort zone. If you need more clarification about using the 4-7-8 breathing method or any other breathing exercise, consider obtaining advice from a trained prenatal yoga teacher or healthcare practitioner.

CHAPTER FOUR

Gentle Yoga Poses during the First Trimester

Gentle yoga postures throughout the first trimester of pregnancy may help you keep active, ease pain, and support your growing body. Concentrating on safe and comfortable positions is vital, and avoiding deep twists or challenging backbends is critical. Always listen to your body; if you encounter any pain, adjust or skip postures as required. Here are some mild yoga positions ideal for the first trimester of pregnancy:

Cat-Cow Pose (Marjaryasana-Bitilasana)

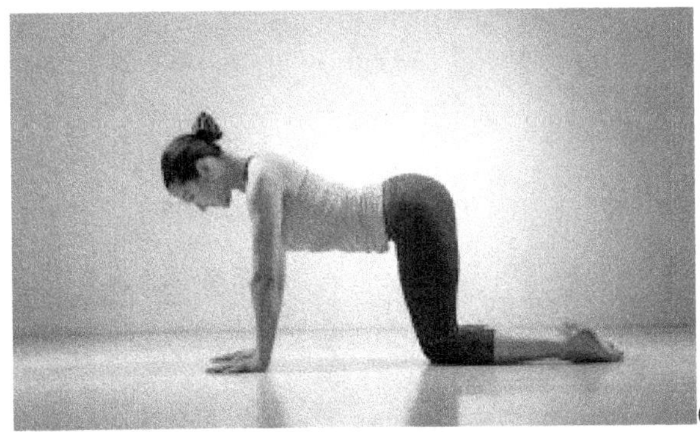

Cat-Cow posture (Marjaryasana-Bitilasana) may be a healthy and safe yoga posture to practice during pregnancy, particularly in the first trimester. This soft, flowing exercise helps to warm up the spine, ease tension, and enhance flexibility. However, there are several adaptations and concerns you should bear in mind to protect your comfort and safety during pregnancy:

Start in Tabletop Position:

- Begin on your hands and knees in a tabletop position.
- Align your wrists beneath your shoulders and your knees under your hips.
- Spread your fingers wide for stability.

Cat Pose (Marjaryasana):

- Inhale as you arch your back softly, elevating your tailbone towards the ceiling.
- Allow your tummy to descend towards the floor, generating a slight curvature in your lower back.
- Lift your head and stare ahead or slightly up without straining your neck.

Cow Pose (Bitilasana):

- Exhale as you go into Cow Pose. Drop your belly towards the floor.
- Pull your tailbone slightly and gradually pull your chest forward, pushing your shoulder blades closer to each other.
- Allow your sight to rise, but avoid overextending your neck.

Flow Between Cat and Cow:

- Inhale, going into Cat Pose with an arched back and elevated tailbone.

- Exhale into Cow Pose with a softly rounded back and elevated chest.
- Continue this flowing movement, syncing your breath with each motion.

Modifications and Considerations:

1. **Maintain a Neutral Spine:** Instead of accentuating the arch and rounding the spine, opt for a more neutral posture. Avoid deep angles or extreme rounding of the back.

2. **Breathe Smoothly:** Focus on breathing smoothly and comfortably throughout the movement. Avoid any breath retention or vigorous Breathing.

3. **Avoid Overstretching:** Avoid overstretching the abdominal region, particularly as your belly expands. Keep the motions moderate and soft.

4. **Use Props:** Placing a cushion or yoga block beneath your hands helps reduce strain on your wrists and give extra support.

5. **Listen to Your Body:** If something seems unpleasant or creates strain, alter or omit the position altogether.

Benefits:

- Cat-Cow Pose helps enhance spinal flexibility and mobility, which may be particularly advantageous when your body changes during pregnancy.
- The slow movement fosters relaxation and helps ease tension in the back and shoulders.

- Cat-Cow Pose maintains a healthy breath pattern and might create a feeling of comfort throughout the first trimester.

Modified Downward Facing Dog (Adho Mukha Svanasana)

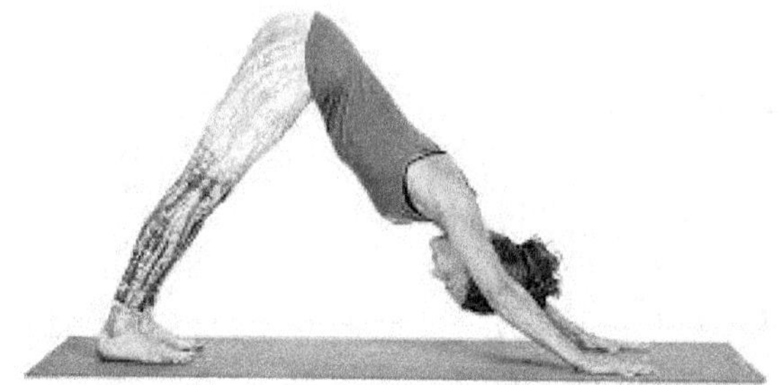

Modified Downward Facing Dog (Adho Mukha Svanasana) may be a safe and pleasant yoga position during pregnancy, especially in the first trimester. However, making specific adaptations is vital to ensure your comfort and safety as your body evolves. Here's how to do a modified version of Downward Facing Dog during pregnancy:

Steps:

1. **Start on All Fours:** Begin in a tabletop posture on your hands and knees. Your wrists should be placed under your shoulders, and your knees should be aligned under your hips.

2. **Walk Your Hands Forward:** Keeping your hips above your knees, slowly walk your hands forward a few inches.

3. **Create a Diagonal Line:** Extend your arms, enabling your body to move into a diagonal line. Your hips should still be above your knees, and your hands should be shoulder-width apart.

4. **Maintain a Flat Back:** Keep your back flat and stretch your spine. Avoid lowering your chest down or rounding your back.

5. **Relax Your Head and Neck:** Let your head hang naturally, relaxing your neck. Your attention might be focused on your mat or slightly ahead.

6. **Bend Your Knees Slightly:** To reduce undue strain on your lower back and to accommodate your increasing tummy, you may bend your knees slightly. This will assist in generating extra room in your torso.

7. **Engage Your Core:** Gently engage your core muscles to stabilize your back and provide stability.

8. **Hold and Breathe:** Stay in this modified posture for a few breaths, concentrating on the stretch in your hamstrings and the elongation of your spine.

9. **Exit the posture:** To come out of the Pose, slowly move your hands back towards your knees, returning to a tabletop position.

1. **Bend Your Knees:** Bending your knees is a critical alteration to allow room for your tummy and reduce tension in your lower back.

2. **Use Props:** Placing blocks beneath your hands helps decrease strain on your wrists and give extra support.

3. **Comfort is Key:** If anything feels unpleasant or causes discomfort, get out of the posture. Listen to your body and practice inside your comfort zone.

Benefits:

- The modified Downward Facing Dog stretches the hamstrings and calf muscles.
- It may help reduce stress in the back and shoulders.
- This stance increases blood circulation and relaxation.

Supported Triangle Pose (Trikonasana)

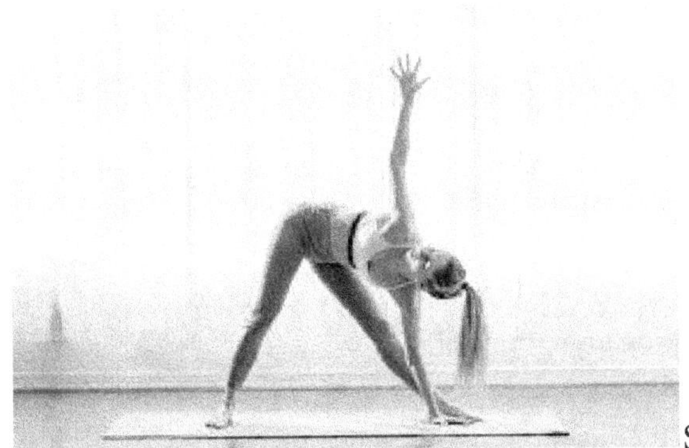

Supported Triangle posture (Trikonasana) may be a good yoga posture to practice during pregnancy, especially in the first trimester. It helps expand the hips and stretch the sides of the body, increasing flexibility and relaxation. However, adaptations are crucial to ensure comfort and safety as your body evolves. Here's how to practice a supported version of Triangle Pose during pregnancy:

Steps:

1. **Use Props:** You'll need a yoga block or a solid cushion to support this modified position.

2. **Stand Tall:** Begin by standing at the top of your mat with your feet comfortably wide apart. Turn your right foot out to the side and your left foot in slightly.

3. **Set the Block:** Hold the yoga block in your right hand and set it on the floor outside your right foot. Adjust the height of the block to a level that feels comfortable for you.

4. **Position Your Feet:** Your front heel should connect with the arch of your back foot. Your feet should be 3 to 4 feet apart, depending on your comfort.

5. **Engage Your Core:** Gently engage your core muscles to stabilize your spine and give stability.

6. **Inhale:** As you inhale, stretch your spine by raising your chest and reaching your left arm towards the sky.

7. **Exhale:** As you exhale, bend at your right hip and tilt your body to the right side. Place your left hand on your left hip.

8. **Rest Your Hand:** Lower your right hand onto the block for support. This will help you maintain balance and reduce strain.

9. **Open Your Chest:** While in the position, concentrate on opening your chest and generating length down the entire side of your body.

10. **Gaze:** If comfortable, turn your head to stare up at your left hand. If this strains your neck, maintain your look ahead or downward.

11. **Hold and Breathe:** Stay in the position for a few breaths, feeling the stretch in your side body and hips.

12. **To Exit:** Inhale as you raise, release your left arm, and return to the beginning position. Turn your feet to face forward.

13. **Perform on the Other Side:** Turn your left foot out and execute the exact instructions on the other side.

Modifications and Considerations:

1. **Use a Higher Block:** If reaching the floor is difficult, use a higher block or position it on its highest level.

2. **Avoid Deep Twisting:** Focus on the stretch in the side body and hips without intensifying the twist. Keep the position comfortable and soft.

Benefits:

- Supported Triangle Pose stretches the sides of the body, hips, and hamstrings.
- It improves excellent posture and flexibility.
- The position may assist in reducing tension in the lower back and hips.

Supported Warrior II (Virabhadrasana II)

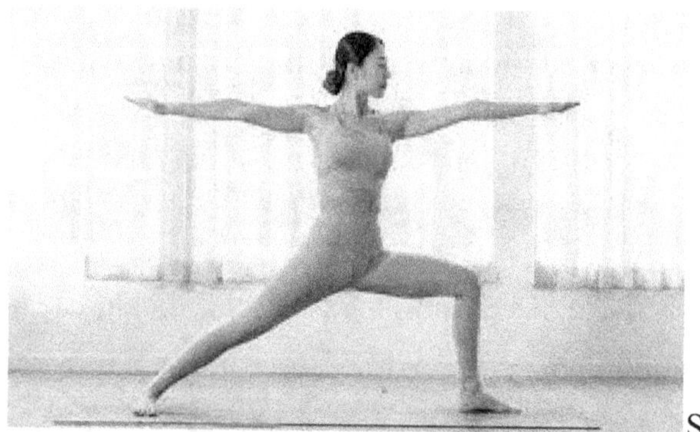

Supported Warrior II (Virabhadrasana II) is a helpful and safe yoga position to practice during pregnancy, particularly in the first trimester. It helps expand the hips, strengthen the legs, and enhance balance and stability. However, adaptations are crucial to ensure comfort and safety as your body evolves. Here's how to practice a supported version of Warrior II during pregnancy:

Steps:

1. **Use Props:** You'll need a yoga block or a solid cushion to support this modified position.

2. **Stand Tall:** Begin by standing at the top of your mat with your feet comfortably wide apart. Turn your right foot out to the side and your left foot in slightly.

3. **Set the Block:** Hold the yoga block in your right hand and put it on the floor inside your right foot. Adjust the height of the block to a level that feels comfortable for you.

4. **Position Your Feet:** Your front heel should connect with the arch of your back foot. Your feet should be 3 to 4 feet apart, depending on your comfort.

5. **Engage Your Core:** Gently engage your core muscles to stabilize your spine and give stability.

6. **Bend Your Front Knee:** As you inhale, bend your right knee, touching your ankle. Ensure that your knee doesn't move past your ankle to avoid strain.

7. **Expand Your Hips:** Gently raise your hips to the side, facing the same direction as your right foot.

8. **Extend Your Arms:** Extend your arms to the sides, parallel to the floor. Your palms may face down or up, depending on your comfort.

9. **Rest Your Left Hand:** Lower your left hand onto the block for support. This will help you maintain balance and reduce strain.

10. **Gaze:** Gently move your head to glance over your right fingers. If this strains your neck, maintain your look ahead or downward.

11. **Hold and Breathe:** Stay in the posture for a few breaths, feeling the stretch in your hips, thighs, and chest.

12. **To Exit:** Inhale as you straighten your front leg, release your left hand, and return to the beginning posture. Turn your feet to face forward.

13. **Perform on the Other Side:** Turn your left foot out and perform the exact instructions on the other side.

1. **Use a Higher Block:** If reaching the floor is difficult, use a higher block or position it on its highest level.
2. **Adjust Your Stance:** If required, you may expand your stance to accommodate your developing tummy.

- Supported Warrior II strengthens and extends the legs, hips, and chest.
- It improves excellent posture, balance, and stability.
- The position may assist in reducing tension in the lower back and hips.

Child's Pose (Balasana)

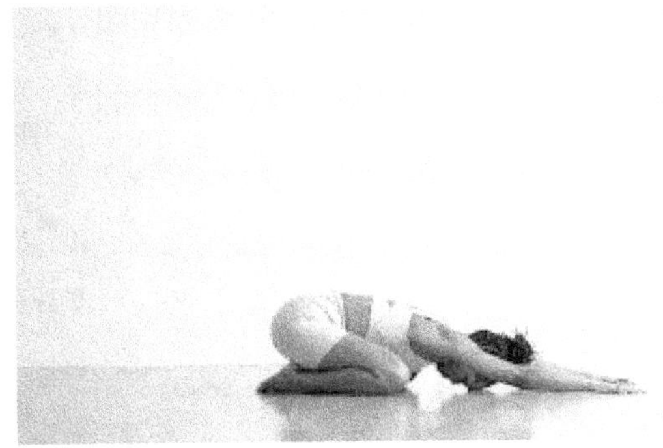

The child's position (Balasana) is a calm and tranquil yoga position that may be particularly useful for pregnant women, especially during the first trimester. It helps eliminate tension, gives a nice stretch, and promotes relaxation. However, making specific alterations is vital to protect your comfort and safety throughout pregnancy. Here's how to practice Child's Pose for pregnant women:

Steps:

1. **Start on Your Mat:** Begin by kneeling on your mat with your big toes touching and your knees apart. Your knees should be broader than your hips to allow room for your tummy.

2. **Sit Back:** Sit back on your heels, allowing your hips to fall towards your heels. If this is unpleasant, insert a pillow or folded blanket between your hips and heels for more support.

3. **Lean Forward:** As inhale, stretch your spine by gently arching your back.

4. **Exhale and Fold:**

- As you exhale, fold forward from your hips.
- Extend your arms forward on the mat, keeping them shoulder-width apart.
- Allow your forehead to rest on the carpet or a cushion if required.

5. **Relax and Breathe:** Relax your whole body. Feel the mild stretch in your lower back and hips. Breathe deeply and pleasantly.

6. **Modify Arm Position:** If extending your arms forward is difficult, you may rest your arms beside your body with your palms facing up.

7. **Hold and Rest:** Stay in this stance as long as you feel comfortable. It's a peaceful stance, so enjoy the tranquillity.

8. **To Exit:** Slowly move your hands back towards your body to come out of the stance. Inhale as you climb back up to a kneeling posture.

Modifications and Considerations:

1. **Use Props:** Place a pillow or folded blanket beneath your hips if sitting back on your heels creates pain. You may also lay a pad or bolster beneath your forehead for support during the forward fold.

2. **Knee Comfort:** If your knees are sensitive, fold a blanket or place a pillow beneath your knees for additional cushioning.

- Child's Pose gives a mild stretch for the hips, thighs, and lower back.
- It creates a sensation of relaxation and helps to ease stress and anxiety.
- The posture is peaceful and supportive, making it great when you need a minute of relaxation throughout your yoga practice.

Supported Bridge Pose (Setu Bandhasana)

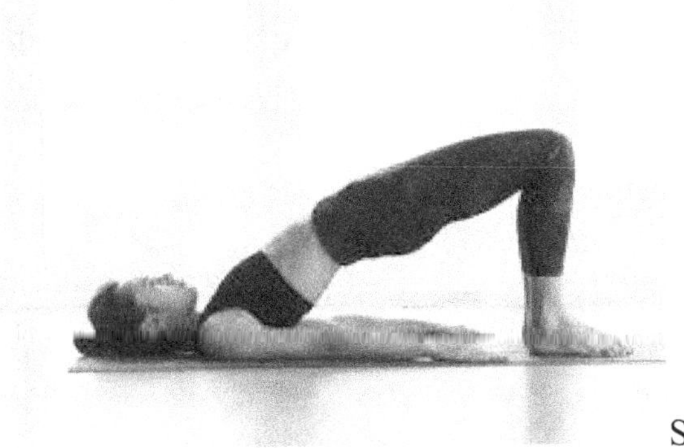

Supported Bridge practice (Setu Bandhasana) may be a calm and restorative yoga practice that promotes comfort and relaxation during pregnancy, particularly in the first trimester. It helps ease lower back ache and opens out the chest and shoulders. However, it's vital to make adaptations to protect your comfort and safety throughout pregnancy. Here's how to practice Supported Bridge Pose for pregnant women:

1. **Gather Props:** You'll need a yoga block or bolster to support this modified posture.

2. **Lie Down:** Start by lying on your back on your mat. Bend your knees and lay your feet flat on the floor, hip-width apart. Your heels should be close to your sitting bones.

3. **Place the Prop:**
- Hold the yoga block or bolster in your hands.
- Gently raise your hips off the ground and slip the prop beneath your sacrum (the bony region at the base of your spine).
- Adjust the support height to a level that feels comfortable for you.

4. **Adjust Your Feet:** Your feet should stay hip-width apart and parallel. Keep your arms relaxed at your sides.

5. **Relax and Breathe:** Allow your body to relax into the support of the prop. Close your eyes and take calm, deep breaths. Feel your chest expanding and your lower back relaxing.

6. **Stay Comfortable:** If you suffer any pain or strain, you may alter the height of the prop or remove it entirely.

7. **Hold and Rest:** Stay in this supported posture for a few breaths or as long as you feel comfortable and restful.

8. **To Exit:** Gently push your feet onto the floor and raise your hips to remove the prop. Lower your hips back down to the mat.

Modifications and Considerations:

- **Use a Higher Prop:** If the prop seems too low, you may use a higher block or bolster to guarantee comfort and support.
- **Avoid Overextension:** While the chest is expanding, avoid overextending your spine. Keep the stretch soft and supportive.

Benefits:

- Supported Bridge Pose reduces stress in the lower back and relieves pain.
- It opens out the chest and shoulders, promoting improved posture.
- The position delivers a sensation of relaxation and healing.

Legs-Up-the-Wall Pose (Viparita Karani)

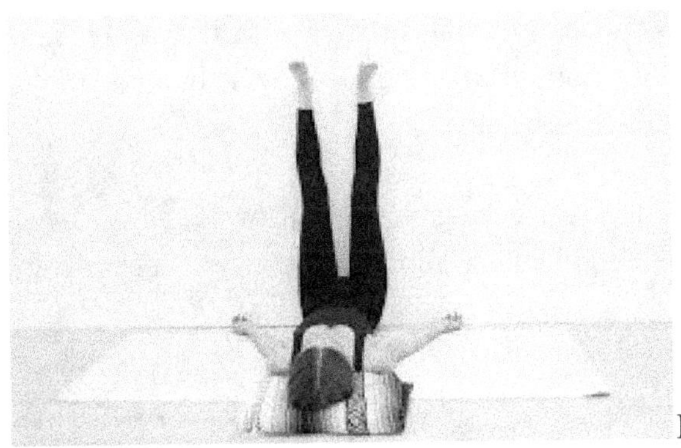

Legs-Up-the-Wall practice (Viparita Karani) may be a relaxing and helpful yoga practice for pregnant women, particularly during the first trimester. It helps decrease oedema in the legs, reduce tiredness, and induce relaxation. However, there are a few adaptations and precautions to assure your comfort and safety throughout pregnancy. Here's how to practice Legs-Up-the-Wall Pose for pregnant women:

Steps:

1. **Prepare Your Space:** Find a clean wall place to perform the position efficiently. You may also use a pillow, folded blanket, or bolster for further support.

2. **Sit Sideways:** Begin by sitting sideways on the floor with your hip contacting the wall. Keep your knees bent and your feet on the floor.

3. **Swing Your Legs Up:** Gently lay down on your back while swinging your legs up the wall. Your sitting bones should approach near the border.

4. **Adjust Distance:** Scoot your hips closer or further away from the wall to reach a comfortable distance. Your body and legs should make a 90-degree angle.

5. **Use Props:** If you experience pain in your lower back or hips, you may lay a folded blanket, pillow, or bolster beneath your hips for support.

6. **Relax and Breathe:**
- Allow your arms to rest comfortably at your sides with your palms facing up.

- Close your eyes and take calm, deep breaths.
- Focus on the sense of relaxation and the mild stretch in your legs.

7. **Stay Comfortable:** If you encounter any pain or strain, you may alter the distance from the wall, tweak the support under your hips, or insert a pillow under your head for increased comfort.

8. **Hold and Rest:** Stay in this supported posture for several minutes, allowing your body to relax and release tension.

9. **To Exit:** To come out of the posture, softly bend your knees and roll to one side. Use your hands to support yourself as you sit up.

Modifications and Considerations:

1. **Use Props:** Props may give extra support and comfort, particularly if you experience stiffness in your lower back or hips.

2. **Avoid Overstretching:** Keep the stretch mild. You should not feel any tension or stiffness in your hamstrings or lower back.

3. **Breathing:** Focus on calm, deep breaths to increase relaxation and awareness during the position.

- Legs-Up-the-Wall Pose promotes blood circulation and helps minimize swelling in the legs and feet, which may be frequent during pregnancy.
- It promotes relaxation and may be especially effective for relieving weariness and stress.
- The posture delivers a sensation of grounding and renewal, making it an excellent alternative for times of self-care.

CHAPTER FIVE

Building Strength and Flexibility in the Second Trimester

Building strength and flexibility throughout the second trimester of pregnancy is vital for supporting your growing body and preparing for delivery. However, it's necessary to approach workouts and yoga positions with prudence and make suitable changes.

Triangle Pose (Trikonasana)

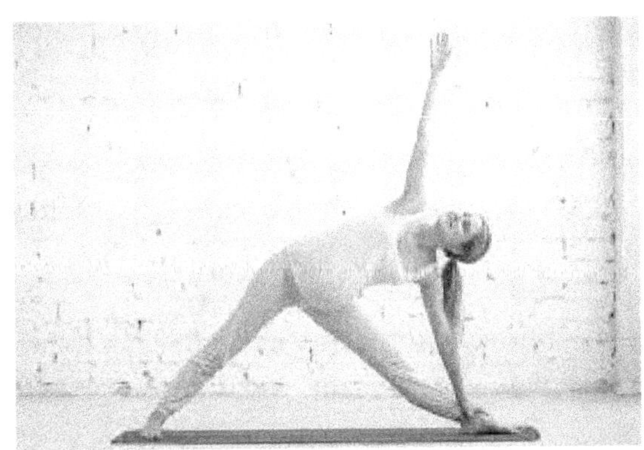

Triangle Pose (Trikonasana) may be performed throughout pregnancy with specific adjustments to ensure comfort and safety. This position helps extend the sides of the body, expand the hips, and develop balance. Here's how to practice Triangle Pose during pregnancy:

Steps:

1. **Start in a Wide Stance:** Stand at the top of your mat with your feet wider than hip-width apart.

2. **Turn Your Foot:** Turn your right foot 90 degrees so your toes point to the mat's top. Your left foot might be slightly turned in.

3. **Stretch Your Arms:** Inhale and stretch your arms to the sides at shoulder height, palms facing down.

4. **Shift Your Hips:** Exhale as you shift your hips to the right and bend at your right hip, extending your right hand toward your right shin, ankle, or a block placed on the floor. Your left arm stretches up toward the ceiling.

5. **Keep Your Chest Open:** Avoid compressing your chest. Instead, concentrate on keeping your chest open and your torso stretched.

6. **Gaze:** Gently turn your head to gaze up at your left hand. If this strains your neck, maintain your look ahead or downward.

7. **Stay Stable:** Keep your weight equally distributed between both feet. Engage your core muscles to support your posture.

8. **Hold and Breathe:** Stay in the posture for a few breaths, feeling the stretch down the right side of your body.

9. **To Exit:** Inhale as you elevate your body, release your left arm, and return to standing. Turn your feet to face forward.

10. **Perform on the Other Side:** Turn your left foot out and perform the exact instructions on the other side.

Modifications and Considerations:

1. **Stance Width:** If your balance is impaired, you may broaden your stance somewhat for increased stability.
2. **Lessen Your Pose:** If your range of motion is restricted or you experience pain, lessen the space between your feet.
3. **Use Props:** If you can't comfortably reach the floor, use a yoga block to support your hand or lay your hand on your shin.
4. **Avoid Deep Bending:** During pregnancy, avoid deep bending or overstretching. Focus on a moderate stretch rather than attempting to touch the ground.

Benefits:

- The triangle Pose helps stretch the sides of the body and enhances flexibility.
- It expands the hips and improves improved posture.
- The posture may help reduce stress and soreness in the lower back and hips.

Tree Pose (Vrikshasana)

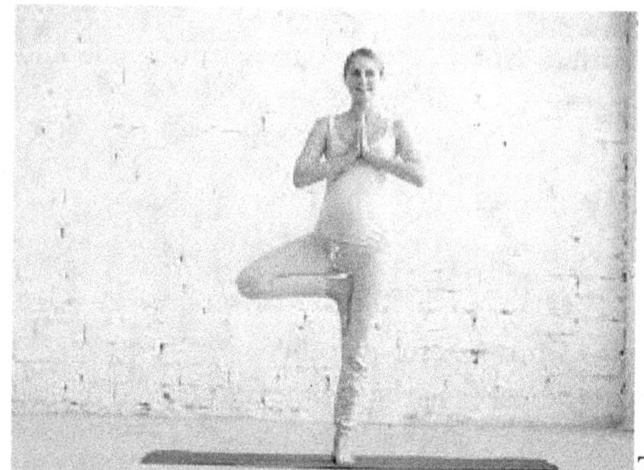

Tree Pose (Vrikshasana) may be performed with certain adjustments during pregnancy to increase balance and attention while preserving stability. This position strengthens the legs and raises awareness. Here's how to practice Tree Pose during pregnancy:

Steps:

1. **Stand Tall:** Begin by standing at the top of your mat with your feet hip-width apart and your arms at your sides.

2. **Shift Your Weight:** Shift your weight onto your left foot. Keep your left leg solid and anchored.

3. **Place Your Foot:** Lift your right foot and place the sole of your right foot on your left inner thigh. Avoid putting it directly on the knee joint; instead, place it above or below the knee.

4. **Hands:** You may maintain your hands at your heart centre in a prayer stance, stretch them aloft, or rest them on your hips.

5. **Find Balance:** Focus on a point before you to maintain balance. Engage your core muscles to support your posture.

6. **Hold and Breathe:** Stay in the position for a few breaths, establishing your balance and maintaining stability.

7. **To Exit:** Gently release your right foot and return it to the floor. Shake out your leg if required.

8. **Perform on the Other Side:** Shift your weight onto your right foot and perform the exact instructions on the other side.

Modifications and Considerations:

1. **Foot Placement:** If resting your foot on your inner thigh is unpleasant, you may place it against your calf or ankle for improved stability.
2. **Use Support:** If you're having problems balancing, stand near a wall or chair for support. Lightly contact the wall with your fingers for balance.

Benefits:

- Tree Pose increases balance and stability, which may be helpful during pregnancy when your centre of gravity moves.
- It strengthens the muscles in your legs and hips.
- The stance fosters attention and focus.

Wide-Legged Forward Fold (Prasarita Padottanasana)

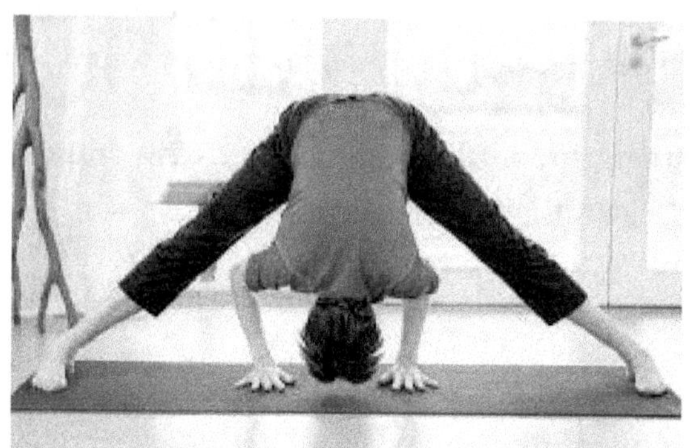

Wide-Legged Forward Fold (Prasarita Padottanasana) may be a helpful yoga position during pregnancy, mainly with adjustments to ensure comfort and safety. This posture helps stretch the hamstrings, inner thighs, and lower back, encouraging relaxation and preserving flexibility. Here's how to practice the Wide-Legged Forward Fold during pregnancy:

Steps:

1. **Start in a Wide Stance:** Stand at the top of your mat with your feet wide apart. Your feet should be broader than hip-width, and your toes may be slightly bent inward.

2. **Engage Your Core:** Gently engage your core muscles to support your lower back and maintain stability.

3. **Inhale and extend:** As you inhale, raise your spine by lifting your chest and facing ahead.

4. **Exhale and Fold:** As you exhale, bend your hips and fold forward. Keep your back flat and preserve a long spine.

5. **Place Your Hands:** Place your hands on the floor beneath your shoulders. Your fingers might point forward or slightly turned in.

6. **Gaze:** Look down towards the floor or slightly forward to maintain your neck straight with your spine.

7. **Bend Your Knees Slightly:** To reduce tension on your lower back and accommodate your developing tummy, you may bend your knees slightly.

8. **Use Support:** Place yoga blocks or props beneath your hands to support your upper body if you can't comfortably reach the floor.

9. **Relax and Breathe:** Allow your head to hang down naturally, and take calm, deep breaths. Feel the stretch in your hamstrings, inner thighs, and lower back.

10. **Hold and Breathe:** Stay in the posture for several breaths, letting your body relax into the stretch.

11. **To Exit:** To come out of the posture, engage your core muscles, bend your knees, and gently raise back up to a standing position.

Modifications and Considerations:

1. **Use Props:** Yoga blocks, props, or a chair might give support if you can't comfortably reach the floor.
2. **Adjust Your Stance:** Widen or narrow your stance depending on your comfort. Make sure your feet are parallel to each other.

Benefits:

- Wide-Legged Forward Fold stretches the hamstrings, inner thighs, and lower back.
- It may help reduce stress in the back and encourage relaxation.
- The posture increases blood circulation and helps preserve flexibility.

Gentle Seated Spinal Twists

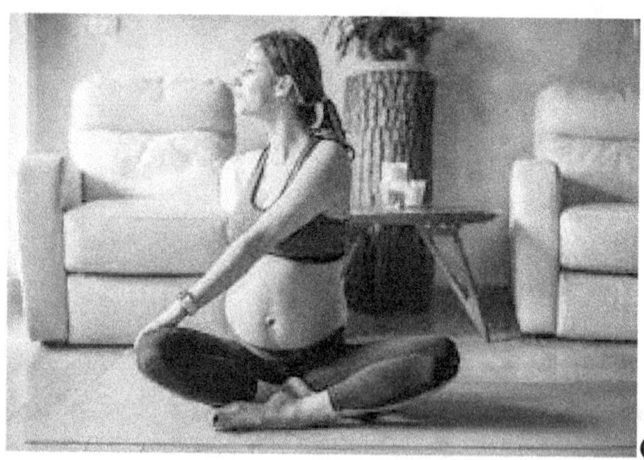

Gentle sitting spinal twists might be an excellent approach to reduce stress and preserve spinal mobility during pregnancy. However, executing these twists carefully and making adaptations to protect your comfort and safety is vital. Here's how to perform mild sitting spinal twists during pregnancy:

Steps:

1. **Start in a Comfortable Seat:** Sit on the floor with your legs in front of you. If required, you may sit on a cushion or folded blanket to raise your hips.

2. **Bend One Knee:** Bend your right knee and put the sole of your right foot on the floor near your left thigh.

3. **Gently Twist:** Inhale to stretch your spine, and as you exhale, gently twist to the right. Place your right hand behind you on the floor for support.

4. **Hold the Twist:** Place your left elbow on the outside of your right knee, gently guiding the twist. Alternatively, lay your left hand on your right thigh.

5. **Keep Your Spine Tall:** Avoid rounding your back. Instead, envision stretching your spine as you twist.

6. **Gaze:** Look over your right shoulder, but avoid over-twisting or straining your neck.

7. **Breathe:** Take calm, deep breaths while you hold the twist. Inhale to extend, and exhale to deepen the twist somewhat.

8. **To Release:** Inhale as you gently come out of the twist. Extend your right leg and sit tall.

9. **Switch Sides:** Repeat the twist on the opposite Side by bending your left leg and twisting to the left.

Modifications and Considerations:

1. **Knee Comfort:** If your knees are sensitive, lay a cushion or folded blanket beneath your bent knee for more cushioning.
2. **Delicate Twists:** Focus on soft twists originating from your upper back rather than deep twists, including your lower back.

Benefits:

- Gentle sitting spinal twists assist in preserving spinal mobility and reduce stress in the back.
- They help reduce pain in the mid and upper back, which might arise owing to changes in posture during pregnancy.
- The twists assist digestion and give a sensation of calm.

Corpse Pose (Savasana)

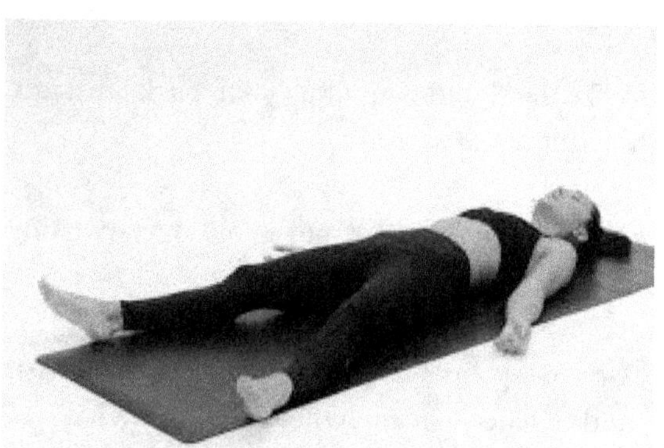

Corpse position (Savasana) is a calming and restorative yoga position that may be performed during pregnancy with specific adjustments to ensure comfort and safety. It's a fantastic method to relieve stress, promote relaxation, and connect with your body and baby. Here's how to practice Corpse Pose during pregnancy:

1. **Prepare Your Space:** Find a pleasant and peaceful area to lay down. You may use cushions, bolsters, or blankets to support your body.

2. **Lie Down:** Lie on your left Side to alleviate strain on the vena cava, a central vein that sends blood back to the heart. Use cushions or pillows to support your head, tummy, and knees.

3. **Relax Your Body:** Allow your body to relax into a comfortable posture. Close your eyes and take a few deep breaths to alleviate stress.

4. **Support Your Head:** Place a pillow or folded blanket beneath your head. You may also use an eye cushion to block out light and increase relaxation.

5. **Support Your Tummy:** Use a cushion or bolster beneath your stomach to give mild support. This may reduce strain on the lower back.

6. **Support Your Knees:** Place a pillow or blanket beneath your knees for increased comfort and relaxation.

7. **Arms and Hands:** Rest your arms beside your body, palms facing up. You may also lay your hands on your tummy for a caring connection.

8. **Breathe:** Take calm, deep breaths. Inhale profoundly and expel thoroughly to encourage relaxation.

9. **Stay in Savasana:** Stay in this supported pose as long as you're comfortable. Aim for at least 5-10 minutes to enable yourself to relax.

Modifications and Considerations:

1. **Left Side Lying:** Lying on your left Side is suggested during pregnancy to enhance blood circulation and minimize strain on the vena cava.
2. **Support Under Belly:** Placing a cushion or bolster under your belly may give comfort and support, mainly as your stomach develops.
3. **Comfort is Key:** Use as many pillows, blankets, and supports as you need to make yourself comfortable.

Benefits:

- Corpse Pose offers profound relaxation and decreases tension.
- It may ease weariness and give you a peaceful area to connect with your body and baby.
- The supported posture may reduce strain on the lower back and give comfort during pregnancy.

Prenatal Sun Salutations

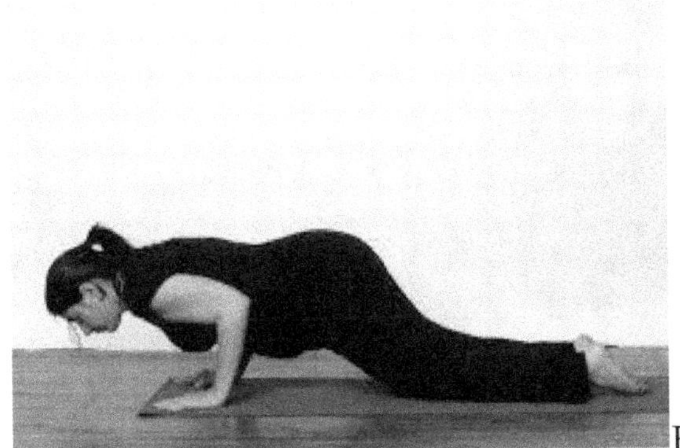

Prenatal Sun Salutations are modified versions of the classic Sun Salutations (Surya Namaskar) that are mainly developed to fit the changing demands of pregnant women. They assist in enhancing circulation, preserving strength, and increasing flexibility while considering the safety and comfort of both the mother and the developing baby. Here's a short series of Prenatal Sun Salutations:

Modified Prenatal Sun Salutation:

Note: *Make sure to warm up your body before doing this pattern. If you're new to yoga or pregnant fitness, try practising under the instruction of a trained prenatal yoga teacher.*

Mountain Pose (Tadasana):

- Stand at the top of your mat with feet hip-width apart.
- Gently rest your hands on your tummy and take a few deep breaths, connecting with your baby.

Modified Forward Fold (Uttanasana):

- Inhale, lift your arms above.
- Exhale, fold forward from your hips and bend your knees slightly if required.
- Rest your hands on your thighs, shins, or a block.

Modified Lunge (Anjaneyasana):

- Inhale, step your right foot back into a lunge stance, keeping your back knee down.
- Lift your chest and lay your hands on your front thigh.
- Hold for a few breaths, feeling the stretch in your hip flexors.

Downward Facing Dog (Adho Mukha Svanasana):

- Exhale, step your left foot back to Downward Facing Dog.
- Keep your knees slightly bent and your hips elevated.
- Press onto your hands and feet, stretching your spine.

Plank Pose (Phalakasana):

- Inhale, move forward to a modified Plank Pose with your knees down.
- Align your shoulders over your wrists and engage your core.

Knees-Chest-Chin Pose:

- Lower your knees, chest, and chin to the floor as you exhale.

- Inhale, slide into Cobra Pose, keeping your hips on the ground.
- Press your hands into the floor and elevate your chest, stretching your spine.

- Exhale, push your hips back to Child's Pose, resting on your thighs.
- Extend your arms forward or beside your body, depending on your comfort.

- Inhale, come back up to Mountain Pose, standing tall with your arms by your sides.
- Repeat the motion on the other Side, stepping the left foot back into a lunge in step 3.

Hip Openers and Gentle Twists

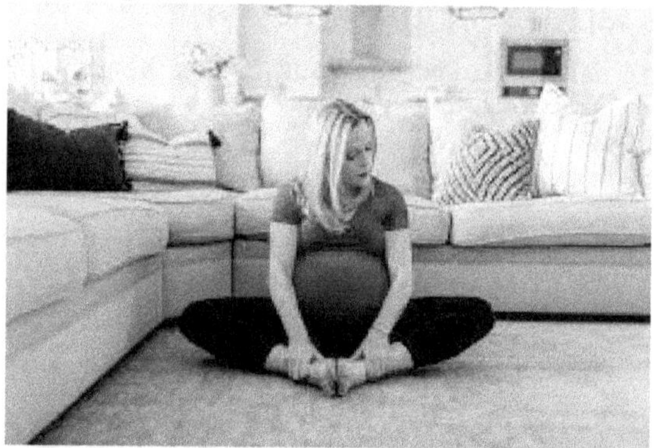

Hip openers and mild twists might be suitable during pregnancy to reduce stress, preserve flexibility, and improve comfort. Here's a sequence that includes hip openers and gentle twists, taking in mind the safety and comfort of pregnant women:

Hip Opener and Gentle Twist Sequence:

Note: *Always warm up your body before doing this pattern.*
Use props like pillows, bolsters, or blankets for further support.
If you're new to yoga or pregnant fitness, try practising under the instruction of a trained prenatal yoga teacher.

Easy Pose with Hip Circles:

- Sit comfortably in Easy Pose (cross-legged stance).
- Gently circle your hips circles and counterclockwise to warm up your hip joints.
- Take deep breaths as you go.

Modified Bound Angle Pose (Baddha Konasana) with Forward Fold:

- Place the soles of your feet together, letting your knees slide out to the sides.
- Hold your feet or ankles with your hands.
- Inhale, stretch your spine, and as you exhale, softly fold forward.
- Support your forehead with a pillow or block.

Gentle Seated Spinal Twist:

- Sit tall and inhale.
- Exhale, twist to the right, resting your left hand on your right knee and your right hand behind you for support.
- Inhale to stretch your spine, and exhale to deepen the twist.
- Gently twist from your upper back while keeping your tummy comfortable.

Modified Pigeon Pose (Eka Pada Rajakapotasana):

- Come onto your hands and knees.
- Bring your right knee forward and position it behind your right wrist.
- Extend your left leg behind you.
- Support your hips with pillows or supports as required.
- Gently fold forward, keeping your spine long.

- Lie on your back with your legs bent and feet flat on the floor.
- Extend your arms out to the sides at shoulder level.
- Exhale, lower your knees to the right, rotating your body to the left.
- Turn your head to the left or maintain it neutral.
- Stay in the twist for a few breaths, experiencing the mild stretch.

Switch Sides:

- Return to the middle and repeat the cycle on the opposing Side.

Remember:

- **Breath:** Maintain calm, deep breaths throughout the routine.
- **Comfort:** Use props to support your body and make the positions comfortable.
- **Gentleness:** Avoid deep stretches and twists. Focus on mild motions.

CHAPTER SIX

Easing Discomfort and Promoting Relaxation in the Third Trimester

Easing pain and fostering relaxation in the third trimester of pregnancy is vital for the well-being of both the mother and the baby. Here are some yoga practices and strategies that might help you accomplish this:

Wall-Supported Downward Facing Dog

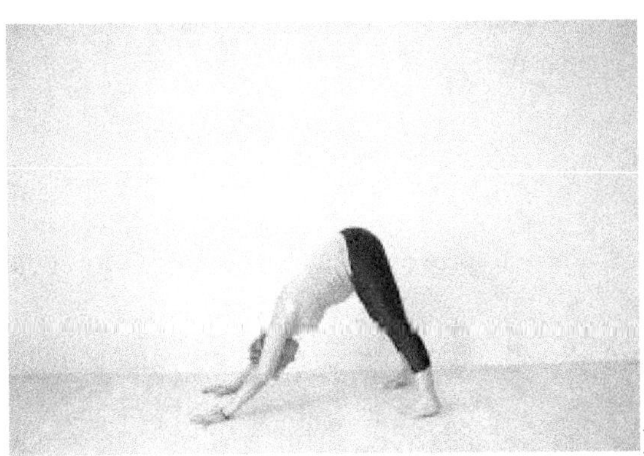During the third trimester of pregnancy, adjusting yoga postures to fit your growing body and maintain safety is crucial. Here's how you may practice a modified Wall-Supported downward-facing dog during the third trimester:

1. Find Your Position:

- Stand facing a wall approximately an arm's length away.
- Place your hands on the wall at shoulder height, with your fingers spread wide.
- Step back a few steps to establish an angle between your body and the wall.

2. Maintain Alignment:

- Keep your feet hip-width apart and parallel to each other.
- Your body should create an inverted V configuration, with your hips higher than your heart.

3. Bend Your Knees:

- Bend your knees slightly to prevent placing too much strain on your lower back.
- This bend will provide more room for your tummy and promote comfort.

4. Gently Stretch:

- Press your hands against the wall, stretching your spine.
- Gently press your hips back to produce a stretch in your hamstrings.

5. Breathe:

- Take slow and deep breaths, allowing your breath to flow freely.
- Focus on relaxing and releasing stress.

6. Avoid Overexertion:

- Do not push yourself too far into the posture. Your comfort is the focus.

7. Support and Balance:

- The wall offers support and stability, letting you experience the advantages of the stretch without strain.

Benefits:

- The modified Wall-Supported downward-facing dog may help reduce back pain by stretching the hamstrings and reducing tension in the spine.
- The wall support guarantees stability and decreases the chance of falling or losing balance.
- Moderate inversion may improve relaxation and enhance blood circulation.

Seated Forward Fold (Paschimottanasana) with Support

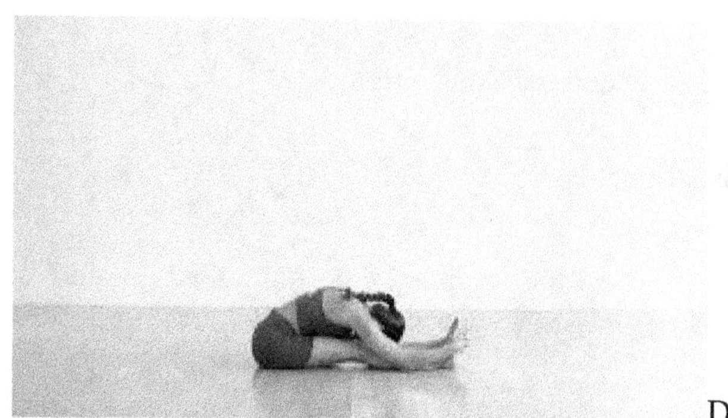

During the third trimester of pregnancy, practising yoga with adjustments is vital to maintain comfort and safety. Here's how you may perform a modified Seated Forward Fold (Paschimottanasana) with assistance at this stage:

Modified Seated Forward Fold with Support:

1. **Find Your Comfortable Seat:**

   - Sit on a pillow or folded blanket to lift your hips slightly. This might give extra room for your belly.

2. **Leg Position:**

   - Extend your legs in front of you, keeping them comfortably apart. Flex your feet to stimulate your leg muscles.

3. **Use Props for Support:**

- Place pillows, bolsters, or folded blankets on your legs. These will support you when you fold inward and reduce pressure on your tummy.

4. **Inhale and Lengthen:**

- Inhale and stretch your spine, sitting tall.

5. **Exhale and Fold Gently:**

- As you exhale, start to fold forward from your hips.
- Support your upper body with the supports you've put on your legs. Allow your head to relax.

6. **Breathe and Relax:**

- Take calm, deep breaths while you remain in the stance.
- Focus on relaxing and releasing any tightness in your back and hamstrings.

7. **Avoid Overstretching:**

- It's crucial not to overstretch. Your tummy could restrict how far you can fold, and that's alright.

8. **Stay Comfortable:**

- The idea is to find a comfortable stretch, not to drive oneself into a deep fold.

Benefits:

- This modified Seated Forward Fold helps stretch the back of your body, particularly the spine, hamstrings, and lower back.
- Using supports and lifting your hips makes the posture more accessible and pleasant.
- Deep breathing during the position may improve relaxation and alleviate tension.

Modified Child's Pose (Balasana) with Props

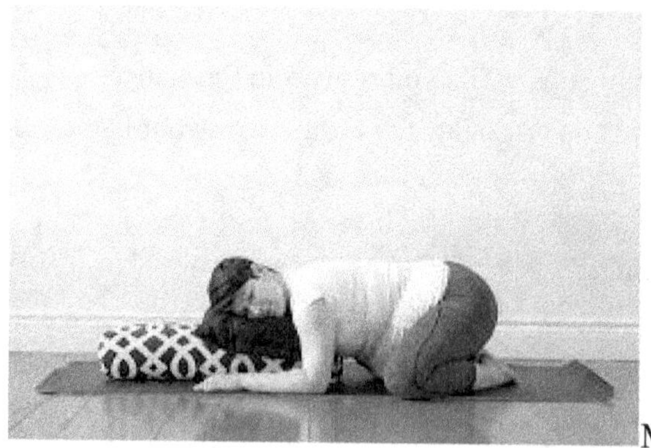

Modified Child's Pose (Balasana) with support may be a fantastic approach to achieve comfort and relaxation during the third trimester of pregnancy. Here's how to practice this stance with modifications:

1. **Gather Your Props:**

   - You'll need a bolster, pillows, or folded blankets to support your body.

2. **Kneel:**

   - Begin by kneeling on the floor. You may tuck a pillow or blanket beneath your knees for added support.

3. **Leg Position:**

   - Bring your knees apart, creating room for your tummy. Your big toes may touch, enabling your knees to expand.

4. **Place the Props:**

   - Place the bolster or cushions in front of you, parallel to your thighs.

5. **Fold Forward:**

   - Slowly lower your upper body onto the supports, allowing your tummy to rest comfortably between your legs.

6. **Head and Arms:**
   - Extend your arms ahead or beside the props. Rest your forehead on the pillow or blanket to support your head.

7. Relax and Breathe:

- Close your eyes and take calm, deep breaths.
- Feel the mild stretch in your back and enjoy the relaxation.

8. Stay as Long as Comfortable:

- Spend several minutes in this supported stance, releasing tension and achieving relaxation.

Benefits:

- The modified Child's Pose with props gives a supportive and pleasant technique to stretch your back, hips, and thighs.
- The supports enable you to rest without straining your tummy or back.
- This position may be highly calming and help ease pain connected with pregnancy.

Caution and Consideration:

- If you sense any discomfort, pressure, or pain in this posture, come out gently.
- If you have any medical ailments or concerns, check with your healthcare professional before doing yoga postures during pregnancy.

Gentle Standing Forward Fold

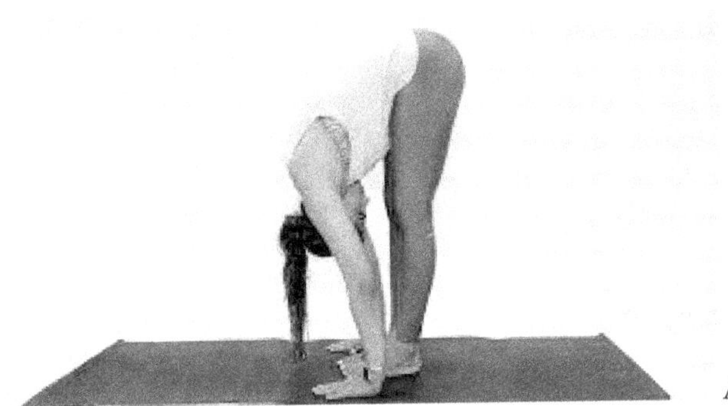

A moderate Standing Forward Fold is a fantastic yoga posture that may bring relaxation, relieve tension in the spine, and deliver a mild stretch to the hamstrings. During the third trimester of pregnancy, it's crucial to adapt postures to fit your developing body. Here's how to practice a modified Gentle Standing Forward Fold at this stage:

Modified Gentle Standing Forward Fold:

1. **Find Your Stance:**
   - Stand with your feet approximately hip-width apart. Keep your feet parallel to each other.

2. **Engage Your Core:**
   - Gently activate your core muscles to support your lower back.
3. **Inhale and Lengthen:**
   - Inhale and stretch your spine, raising your chest higher.

4. **Exhale and Fold:**

- As you exhale, bend your hips and begin to fold forward. Keep a slight bend in your knees.

5. **Support Your Torso:**

- Place your hands on your thighs and shins, or use yoga blocks on the floor for support.

6. **Avoid Overstretching:**

- The aim is not to touch the floor or attain a deep stretch, mainly if your tummy makes it challenging.

7. **Relax Your Head and Neck:**

- Allow your head to hang down naturally. If you're comfortable, you may gently nod yes and no to alleviate neck strain.

8. **Breathe:**

- Take calm and deep breaths while you hold the stance. Inhale to extend your spine, and exhale to relax into the stretch.

9. **Stay Comfortable:**

- Maintain a comfortable stretch without any effort or pain. Feel free to change your posture or props as required.

10. **To Come Up:**

- Inhale and use your core muscles as you gently raise back to a standing posture.

Benefits:

- The modified Standing Forward Fold delivers a mild stretch to the hamstrings, lower back, and spine.

- It stimulates relaxation and may help alleviate tension in the upper body.
- This position stimulates blood circulation and might produce a sensation of tranquillity.

- If you sense any pain or tension, gently leave the posture.
- As with any position during pregnancy, ask your healthcare professional before practising yoga.
-

Supported Bridge Pose (Setu Bandhasana) with Props

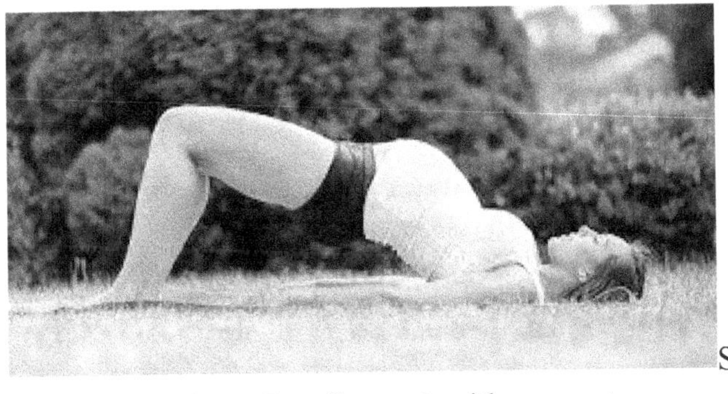

Supported Bridge Pose (Setu Bandhasana) with supports may promote comfort and relaxation during the third trimester of pregnancy. Here's how to practice a modified version of Supported Bridge Pose with props:

1. **Gather Your Props:**
   - You'll need a bolster, pillows, or folded blankets for support.

2. **Set Up Your Space:**
   - Find a comfortable location on your mat or a soft surface.

3. **Lie Down:**
   - Lie on your back with your knees bent and your feet flat on the floor, hip-width apart.

4. **Position the Props:**
   - Place the bolster or cushions horizontally beneath your sacrum (the bony region at the base of your spine). The props should give support without creating pain.

5. **Engage Your Core:**
   - Gently activate your core muscles to support your spine and stabilize your pelvis.

6. **Lift Your Hips:**
   - Inhale as you gently raise your hips off the floor and shift your body to rest on the props.
   - The supports should gently cradle your lower back and hips.

7. **Adjust the Props:**
   - If desired, you may modify the height or location of the props to get the most comfortable support.

8. **Relax and Breathe:**
   - Allow your body to relax into the supported posture.
   - Rest your arms by your sides or on your belly. Close your eyes and take calm, deep breaths.

9. **Stay in the Pose:**
   - Hold the posture for many breaths or as long as it feels comfortable.

10. **To Come Down:**
   - Exhale and gradually drop your hips back down to the floor.

   - The modified Supported Bridge Pose delivers a mild stretch to the chest, shoulders, and hips.
   - Using props supports the lower back and pelvis, facilitating relaxation and minimizing strain on the spine.
   - This position may help decrease lower back stiffness prevalent during the third trimester.

   - If you feel any pain or tension, gently leave the posture.
   - Always check your healthcare provider before doing yoga during pregnancy.

Cat-Cow Pose (Marjaryasana-Bitilasana) on All Fours

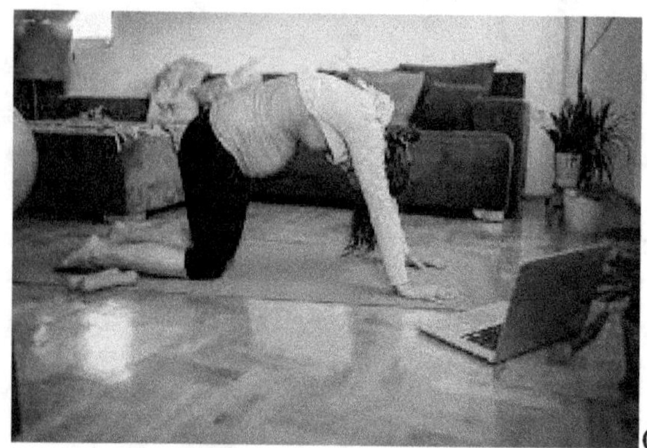Cat-Cow Pose (Marjaryasana-Bitilasana) on all fours may be tailored to the demands of your changing body throughout the third trimester of pregnancy. This simple exercise helps alleviate tension in the spine and develops flexibility. Here's how to practice a modified version of Cat-Cow Pose at this stage:

Modified Cat-Cow Pose on All Fours - Third Trimester:

1. **Get into Position:**
   - Start on your hands and knees, positioning your wrists under your shoulders and your knees under your hips.
   - Spread your fingers wide and push your palms into the mat for support.

2. **Engage Your Core:**
   - Gently activate your core muscles to stabilize your spine and give stability.

3. **Cow Pose (Bitilasana):**
   - Inhale as you arch your back, softly sinking your belly towards the floor. Ascend your tailbone and head, enabling your sight to ascend without straining your neck.
   - This easy backbend expands your chest and extends your tummy.

4. **Cat Pose (Marjaryasana):**
   - Exhale as you circle your back, tucking your tailbone and chin into your chest.
   - Imagine softly holding your baby's tummy as you circle your spine.

5. **Move Mindfully:**
   - Continue to move between Cow and Cat Poses, connecting each movement with your breath.
   - Focus on the flow of the movement and the feelings in your spine.

6. **Tailor the Movement:**
   - As your belly develops, your range of motion may be reduced. Focus on producing a calm, rhythmic flow rather than severe stretches.

7. **Breathe Deeply:**
   - Take slow and deep breaths as you progress through the positions, letting your breath guide your movement.

   - The modified Cat-Cow Pose helps release tension in the spine and expands the chest.
   - This technique softly stretches the abdominal muscles and maintains healthy mobility in the spine.
   - The exercise develops attention and connection with your evolving body.

   - Avoid over-arching or over-rounding your back. Keep the motions soft and controlled.
   - If you suffer any pain or strain, adapt the motions appropriately.
   - Always check your healthcare provider before doing yoga during pregnancy.

Gentle Hip Circles in a Wide-Legged Stance

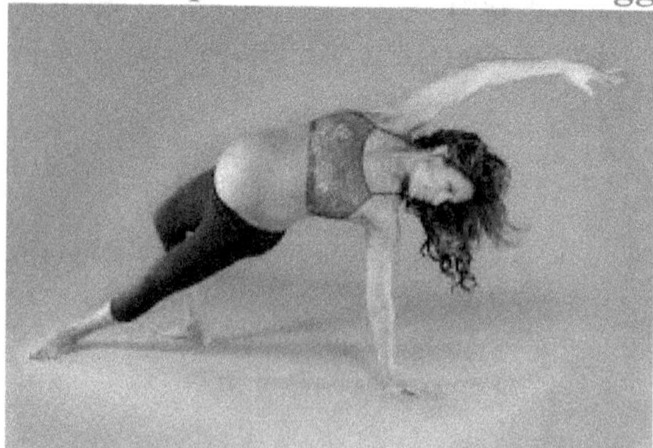

Gentle hip circles in a wide-legged stance may be beneficial during the third trimester of pregnancy to reduce hip stiffness and develop flexibility. Here's how you may alter this dance for the third trimester:

Gentle Hip Circles in a Wide-Legged Stance - Third Trimester:

1. **Find Your Stance:**
   - Stand in the middle of your mat with your feet comfortably wider than hip-width apart. Toes may be slightly bent outward.

2. **Engage Your Core:**
   - Gently engage your core muscles to stabilize and support your lower back.

3. **Hands for Balance:**
   - Place your hands on your hips, or you may rest them softly on your thighs for balance.

4. **Start the Circles:**
   - Inhale as you move your hips to the right Side, producing a circular motion with your hips.
   - As you exhale, repeat the circle by rotating your hips back, to the left, and then forward.

5. **Mindful Movement:**
   - Coordinate your breath with the action. Inhale as you rotate your hips to one Side, and exhale as you complete the circle.

6. **Switch Direction:**
   - After a few rounds in one direction, switch to circling in the opposing way.

7. **Gentle and Fluid:**
   - Keep the movement mild and smooth. Avoid any sudden or violent moves.

8. **Listen to Your Body:**
   - If you suffer any pain or tension, make the circles smaller or slow down the action.

Benefits:
   - Gentle hip circles help ease hip strain and stiffness, which are prevalent throughout the third trimester.
   - The action enhances the flexibility of the hip joints and promotes relaxation.

Caution and Consideration:
   - As you approach your due date, be cautious of your balance and stability. You can practice beside a wall or a hard surface for support.
   - Always check your healthcare provider before doing yoga during pregnancy.

Corpse Pose (Savasana) with Support

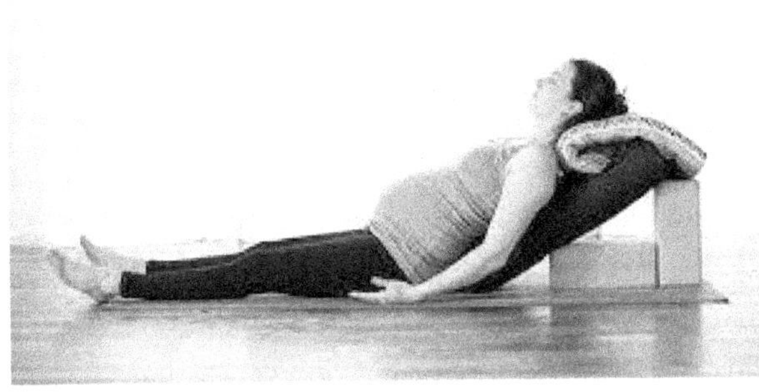

With assistance, corpse Pose (Savasana) is a fantastic technique to relax and revitalize during the third trimester of pregnancy. Here's how you may practice a modified form of Savasana with supporting props:

Modified Corpse Pose with Support - Third Trimester:

1. **Gather Your Props:**
   - You'll need pillows, cushions, or bolsters to support your body in a reclining posture.

2. **Lie Down Comfortably:**
   - Find a comfortable location on your mat or a soft surface.

3. **Position Your Props:**
   - Place one or two pillows, bolsters, or cushions beneath your head and upper back. The props should support your head and enable you to recline comfortably.

4. **Bend Your Knees:**
   - Bend your knees and lay your feet flat on the floor, hip-width apart.

5. **Use a Prop for Belly Support:**
   - If desired, lay a pillow or cushion beneath your tummy to support the weight and provide a sensation of relaxation.

6. **Relax Your Arms:**
   - Allow your arms to rest beside your body, with your palms facing up.

7. **Close Your Eyes:**
   - Close your eyes to limit external disturbances and enhance inner calm.

8. **Focus on Your Breath:**
   - Pay attention to your breath as you inhale and exhale freely. Let your breath be gentle and easy.

9. **Release Tension:**
   - Mentally scan your body and intentionally release any places of tightness.

10. **Visualize Relaxation:**
   - Imagine each body part getting heavy and sinking into the support underneath you.

11. **Stay in the Pose:**
   - Remain in this supported posture for several minutes, allowing your body to relax entirely.

12. To Come Out:

- When you're ready to emerge from the posture, softly wriggle your fingers and toes to awaken your body. Roll to your Side and take a few breaths before carefully sitting up.

Benefits:

- The modified Corpse Pose with support gives profound relaxation to the whole body.
- Using supports to support your body's weight might ease lower back and hip stiffness.
- This position promotes mental relaxation and may help relieve tension and weariness.

Caution and Consideration:

- Adjust the props or come out of the posture gently if you suffer any difficulty.
- Always check your healthcare provider before doing yoga during pregnancy.

CHAPTER SEVEN

Partner Yoga and Connection with Your Baby

Spouse yoga during pregnancy may be a great way to connect with your spouse and develop a baby. It gives a chance to share the pregnancy experience, encourage relaxation, and establish a feeling of togetherness. Here are a few partner yoga positions that you might practice during pregnancy to develop a connection:

Sitting Back-to-Back Meditation

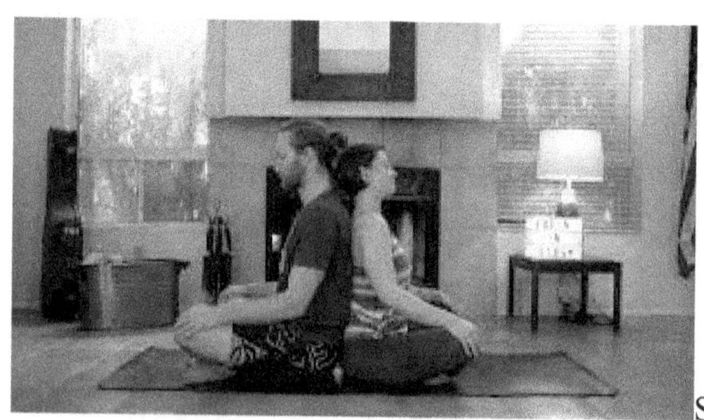

Sitting back-to-back meditation is a simple and profound practice that may help you and your spouse connect, relax, and support one another throughout pregnancy. Here's how you can practice sitting back-to-back meditation:

1. **Find a Comfortable Space:**

   - Choose a peaceful and comfortable area where you and your spouse can sit.

2. **Sit Back-to-Back:**
   - Sit comfortably on the floor with your legs crossed or in a comfortable sitting posture.
   - Your backs should be touching, providing a soft connection between you and your companion.

3. **Close Your Eyes:**
   - Close your eyes and take a minute to relax within the space.

4. **Focus on Your Breath:**
   - Begin to concentrate your attention on your breath. Notice the natural rhythm of your inhales and exhales.

5. **Sync Your Breaths:**
   - As you both breathe, attempt to sync your breaths with each other.
   - Inhale and exhale simultaneously, allowing your breaths to synchronize.

6. **Feel the Connection:**
   - As you breathe together, you'll naturally feel the soft movement of your partner's back against yours.

- Allow this physical connection to increase your feeling of closeness and support.

7. **Release Tension:**
   - As you continue to breathe, let go of any tension in your body and thoughts.
   - Imagine breathing in good energy and expelling any tension or anxieties.

8. **Stay in the Moment:**
   - Stay in this sitting meditation for a few minutes, allowing the connection and shared breaths to generate a feeling of serenity and harmony.

9. **Ending the Meditation:**
   - Take a few deep breaths together when you're ready to conclude the meditation.
   - Gently open your eyes and take time to savour the sensation.

Benefits:
   - Sitting back-to-back meditation allows you and your partner to feel a sense of presence and connection.
   - Shared breath and physical touch may enhance relaxation and lessen tension.
   - This practice develops a sense of support and togetherness as you begin on the adventure of pregnancy together.

Remember that relationship practices are about mutual respect and comfort. If you're new to meditation or prenatal activities, try practising under the instruction of a professional prenatal yoga instructor or meditation teacher for specific assistance and changes suited to your pregnancy requirements.

Gentle Shoulder and Back Massage

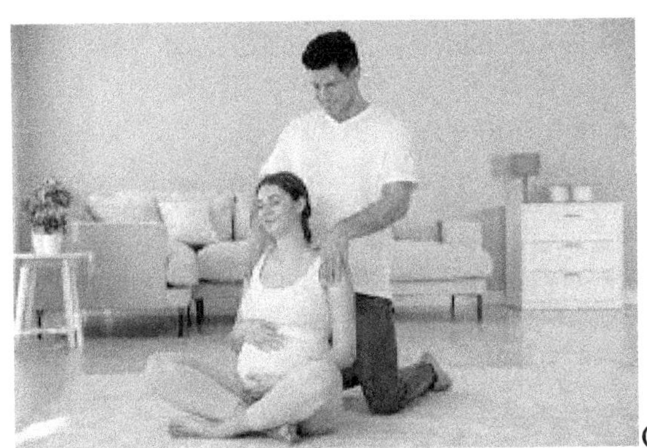

Gentle shoulder and back massages may be a compassionate and bonding activity during pregnancy, bringing relaxation and support to your partner. Here's how you may deliver a gentle shoulder and back massage during the connection time of pregnancy:

1. **Create a Relaxing Environment:**
    * Choose a comfortable and quiet area where you and your companion can sit or lie comfortably.

2. **Use Comfortable Seating:**
    * Sit in a comfortable posture, facing your companion. Your spouse may sit on a cushion or chair.

3. **Start with Relaxation:**
   - Begin the massage by laying your hands softly on your partner's shoulders and taking a few deep breaths together.

4. **Use Gentle Touch:**
   - Use the palms of your hands to offer mild pressure on your partner's shoulders and upper back.

5. **Kneading and Circular Motions:**
   - Use your fingers to knead and gently move your partner's upper back and shoulders.
   - Apply light pressure and modify according to your partner's comfort level.

6. **Move Along the Spine:**
   - Use your fingers to softly trace down the sides of your partner's spine, working upward from the lower back to the shoulders.

7. **Offer Neck Support:**
   - Gently hold your partner's head with both hands, delivering support to the neck. Use your thumbs to make little circular movements at the base of the skull.

8. **Communication:**
   - Throughout the massage, ask your spouse for input on pressure and comfort. Adjust your technique appropriately.

9. **Focus on Relaxation:**
   - Encourage your spouse to relax and let go of any stress while you perform the massage.

10. Be Mindful of Time:

- Spend a few minutes rubbing each region before moving on to the next.

11. Ending the Massage:

- Gradually ease out of the massage with gentle, soft strokes on your partner's back.

12. Express Gratitude:

- End the massage with a soft touch and offer thanks for the chance to give relaxation and support.

Benefits:

- Gentle massages promote relaxation and help alleviate muscular tension.
- The technique fosters a feeling of closeness and care between couples.
- This massage helps generate a pleasant and tranquil atmosphere throughout the connection phase of pregnancy.

Seated Heart-to-Heart Pose

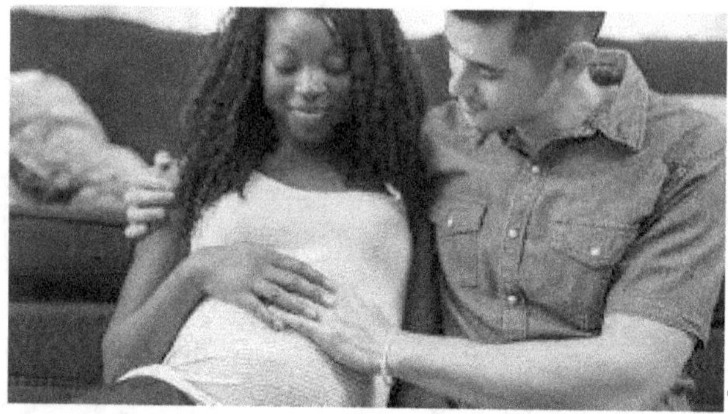

The seated Heart-to-Heart position is a gentle and personal yoga position that may help spouses connect with their developing baby during pregnancy. This stance fosters a feeling of unity and delivers an emotional experience. Here's how you can practice Seated Heart-to-Heart Pose:

1. **Find a Quiet Space:**
    - Choose a peaceful and comfortable area where you and your spouse may sit facing each other.

2. **Sit Comfortably:**
    - Sit on the floor or cushions cross-legged, facing each other.

3. **Knee-to-Knee Connection:**
    - Bring the soles of your feet together, allowing your knees to fall wide towards the sides.

4. **Hold Hands:**
    - Reach out and clasp hands with your companion. Your hands may rest on your partner's knees.

5. **Close Your Eyes:**
   - Close your eyes and take a minute to tune into your breath and the connection between you and your spouse.

6. **Lean Back Gently:**
   - Both lovers may lean back slightly, enabling your hearts to draw closer together.

7. **Connection with Baby:**
   - If you're comfortable, gently put your other hand on your tummy, experiencing the connection with your baby.

8. **Maintain Eye Contact:**
   - Keep your eyes closed or delicate eye contact with your partner, providing a feeling of closeness and connection.

9. **Breathe Together:**
   - Take long, deep breaths together. Inhale and exhale in a coordinated way, enabling your breaths to blend.

10. **Share Your Thoughts:**
    - Use this time to communicate your thoughts, emotions, and intentions with each other and your baby.

11. **Express Love and Gratitude:**
    - Take a minute to express your love and thanks for the trip you're on together.

12. Ending the Pose:

- When you're ready to come out of the stance, softly release your hands and open your eyes.

- Seated Heart-to-Heart Pose develops a profound emotional connection between lovers.
- The posture fosters free conversation and gives a tranquil setting to connect with your kid.
- It fosters calm, trust, and shared purpose throughout the spouse and infant bonding time.

Partner Child's Pose

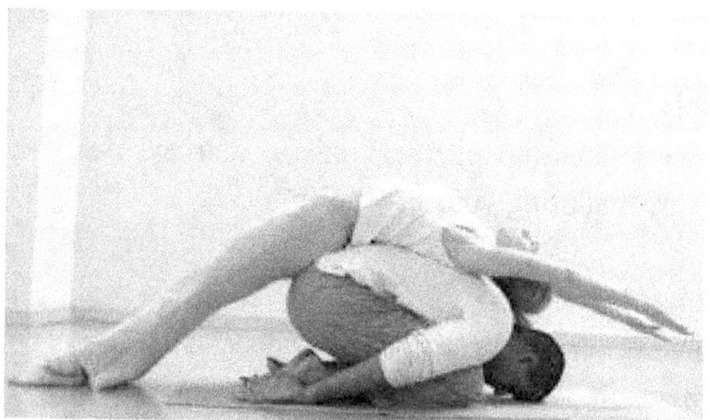

1. Create Space:

- Spread your knees wide apart, allowing enough room for both partners to sit between each other's legs comfortably.

2. **Partner Support:**
   - One person gradually sits back between the other partner's legs, offering a comfortable, relaxing area.

3. **Fold Forward:**
   - The sitting partner leans forward, letting their chest rest on the floor. The arms may be stretched in front or rest beside the torso.

4. **Partner's Hands:**
   - The standing partner might gently lay their hands on the sitting partner's back or shoulders, giving support and comfort.

5. **Breathe Together:**
   - Both couples take calm, deep breaths, generating a shared relaxation and connection.

6. **Support and Nurturing:**
   - The sitting partner may feel the soft pressure and support from the standing partner's hands, producing a sensation of care.

7. **Stay in the Pose:**
   - Stay in the stance for many breaths, making both parties feel connected and relaxed.

8. **Switch Positions:**
   - After a few breaths, exchange positions so that both partners have the chance to experience both roles.

9. **Ending the Pose:**

- When you're ready to come out of the stance, both partners softly relax and sit back.

- Partner Child's Pose gives a comfortable and loving experience between lovers.
- It offers support and relaxation throughout the spouses and infant bonding stage.
- The shared breath and physical touch may generate a magnificent sensation of togetherness and presence.

- Practice concerning each other's comfort and speak honestly.
- Always practice within a range of motion that feels safe and comfortable.

Breathing Together

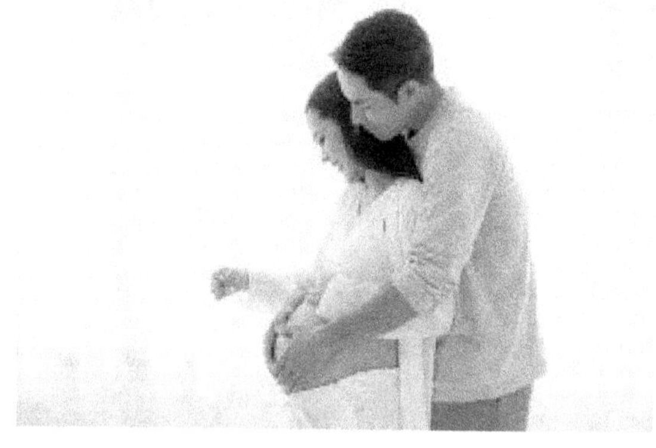

Breathing together is a simple but effective activity that may improve the connection between couples and boost the sensation of closeness throughout the partners and infant connection phase. Here's how you can practice breathing together:

1. **Find a Comfortable Space:**
   - Choose a peaceful and comfortable area where you and your companion can sit or lie comfortably.

2. **Sit Facing Each Other:**
   - Sit in a comfortable posture facing each other. You may sit cross-legged or on pillows.

3. **Hold Hands or Maintain Eye Contact:**
   - Either clasp your hands with your companion or keep gentle eye contact. Choose the option that seems most natural and comfortable for both of you.

4. **Close Your Eyes:**
   - Close your eyes to eliminate extraneous distractions and concentrate on your breath and the connection with your partner.

5. **Begin to Breathe:**
   - Start by taking a few deep breaths together. Inhale deeply through your nose and exhale through your mouth.

6. **Sync Your Breath:**
   - As you breathe, attempt to synchronize your breath with your partner's. Inhale and exhale simultaneously, allowing your breaths to sync.

7. **Feel the Rhythm:**
   - Pay attention to the rhythm of your breathing and your connection with your companion.

8. **Deepen the Connection:**
   - As you continue breathing together, picture your breaths generating a circle of energy between you and your companion.

9. **Set an Intention:**
   - While breathing, make an intention or a good thought for yourself, your spouse, and your kid.

10. **Express Gratitude:**
    - As you finish the exercise, take a minute to express thanks for this shared experience.

11. **Take a Final Breath:**
    - Inhale deeply, hold your breath momentarily and then expel fully.

12. **Open Your Eyes:**
    - Gently open your eyes and take a minute to connect with your companion via your gaze.

- Breathing together fosters synchronization and harmony between lovers.
- It provides a sensation of peace, relaxation, and shared presence.
- The technique increases emotional connection and bonding throughout the couple and infant connection time.

- Be patient and compassionate with each other. Allow the breath to flow naturally and pleasantly.
- This practice might be beneficial if you and your spouse seek times of quiet connection and shared attention throughout pregnancy.

Savasana with Hand Connection

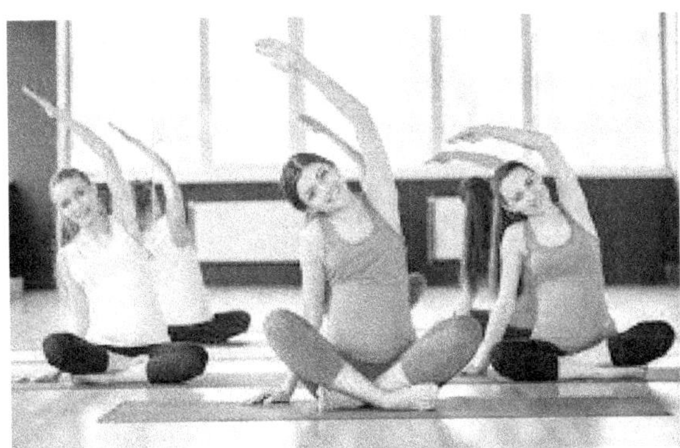

Savasana with hand connection is an excellent method for couples to rest together, build a feeling of contact, and enjoy a tranquil time during the partner and baby connection phase. Here's how you can practice Savasana with hand connection:

1. **Prepare a Comfortable Space:**
   - Set up a calm and comfortable location where you and your spouse may lie down.

2. **Lie Down Comfortably:**
   - Side by Side, lie down on your backs, with a little room between you.

3. **Support Your Head and Neck:**
   - Place a pillow or cushion beneath your head and neck for support. Ensure that your spine is aligned.

4. **Bend Your Knees:**
   - Bend your knees and allow your feet to fall quickly to the sides. Allow your legs to relax.

5. **Hand Connection:**
   - Extend one arm to the Side and have your companion do the same.
   - Reach out and softly clasp hands with your companion, establishing a physical connection between you.

6. **Close Your Eyes:**
   - Close your eyes and take a few deep breaths together to relax into the position.

7. **Relax Your Body:**
   - Allow your whole body to relax into the support of the floor and whatever props you're utilizing.

8. **Sync Your Breaths:**
   - Begin to coordinate your breathing. Inhale deeply collectively and exhale with a sensation of letting go.

9. **Visualize Connection:**
   - As you breathe, envision the energy of your breaths joining and flowing through the space between your hands.

10. **Shared Relaxation:**
    - Let go of any tension and concentrate on the relaxation flowing throughout your body.

11. **Stay in the Pose:**
    - Remain in Savasana with a hand connection for many minutes, letting yourself relax.

12. **Ending the Pose:**
    - To leave the posture, gently release your hands and allow a few minutes to transition.

Benefits:

- With a hand touch, Savasana creates a tremendous sensation of connection and closeness.
- The combined breath and hand touch produce a serene and relaxing experience.

- The exercise encourages calm, emotional connectedness, and a shared presence.

- Be conscious of each other's comfort and make modifications as required.
- If you notice any difficulty, gently change the stance or come out of it.

Sharing Intentions

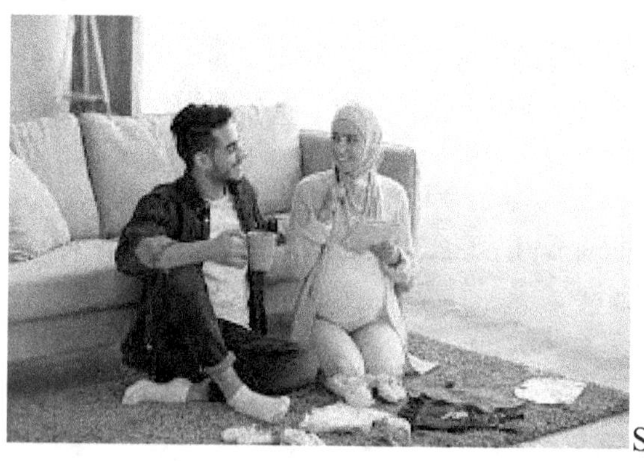

Sharing intentions is a significant ritual that helps couples synchronize their ideas, wishes, and emotions throughout the partners and baby bonding phase. This technique encourages open communication and enhances the bond between teams as they begin the adventure of pregnancy together. Here's how you can practice conveying intentions:

1. **Create a Calm Space:**
   - Find a quiet and comfortable area where you and your spouse may sit facing each other.

2. **Sit Comfortably:**
   - Sit cross-legged or on pillows, facing each other.

3. **Center Yourself:**
   - Close your eyes and take a few deep breaths to focus on yourself.

4. **Hold Hands:**
   - Reach out and clasp hands with your companion, establishing a physical connection.

5. **Set the Intention:**
   - Begin by expressing an aim or idea relevant to your pregnancy journey. This might be a hope, a desire, or a sentiment you'd want to communicate.

6. **Take Turns:**
   - Take turns discussing your objectives. One partner talks while the other listens carefully.

7. **Active Listening:**
   - As your spouse talks, listen with an open heart and without interruption.

8. **No Judgment:**
   - Create a non-judgmental and supportive place where both partners feel secure to express themselves.

9. **Speak from the Heart:**
   - Share your objectives truthfully, coming from your heart.

10. **Express Gratitude:**
    - After each couple discusses their purpose, thank each other for being open and sharing.

11. **Switch Roles:**
    - Once both parties have communicated their objectives, reverse positions and take turns speaking and listening.

12. **Closing the Practice:**
    - After both partners have had the chance to speak, finish the practice with a last moment of handholding and connection.

Benefits:

- Sharing intentions improves open communication and understanding between couples.
- It helps couples to communicate their thoughts and aspirations in a secure and loving setting.
- The exercise improves the sensation of connection and oneness throughout the couple and infant bonding time.

Caution and Consideration:

- Be attentive and present while your spouse is revealing their intentions.
- Approach this exercise with an open heart and a desire to listen and support each other.

CHAPTER EIGHT

Labour Preparation and Pain Management

Breathing Techniques for Labor

Breathing methods are crucial for reducing discomfort, inducing calm, and keeping concentration throughout birth. Different breathing methods help you deal with the different phases of labour. Here are some excellent breathing strategies during delivery:

Slow and Deep Breathing:

- Inhale gently through your nose, extending your abdomen.
- Exhale softly through your mouth, releasing tension and concentrating on relaxation.
- This approach helps you remain calm and concentrated throughout the early stages of labour.

Cleansing Breath:

- Inhale deeply through your nose.
- Exhale powerfully through your lips, generating a "ha" sound.
- This approach may relieve tension and provide a feeling of catharsis.

Modified Panting Breath:
- Inhale deeply through your nose.

- Exhale in short, rapid bursts via your mouth.
- This approach may be practical during the active period of labour to control contractions.

Slow Exhale:

- Inhale deeply through your nose.
- Exhale gently and thoroughly through your mouth.
- This approach promotes calm and helps you concentrate on letting go.

Rhythmic Breathing:

- Inhale for a count of four.
- Exhale for a count of four.
- Maintain this pattern, modifying the counts as required.
- Rhythmic breathing helps you remain focused and stable throughout contractions.

Golden Thread Breath:

- Inhale deeply through your nose.
- Exhale softly and evenly as though you're blowing on a fragile thread.
- This approach develops relaxation and control.

Visualization Breathing:

- Inhale deeply, imagining good energy entering your body.
- Exhale gently, envisioning tension and agony leaving your body.
- Visualization may help you channel your breath and concentrate your thoughts.

- As contractions peak, take calm, deep breaths into the region where you feel the most significant pain.
- Exhale gradually, thinking that you're releasing the stress and discomfort.

Counted Breaths:

- Inhale for a count of three or four.
- Exhale for the exact count.
- Counted breaths give structure and help control your breathing.

Progressive Relaxation Breathing:

- Inhale deeply while tensing your muscles.
- Exhale gently while releasing the tension and allowing your muscles to relax.
- This approach induces relaxation and may assist in easing pain.

It's vital to practice these breathing methods before labour starts so that you're acquainted with them when the time arrives. During delivery, alter the tactics depending on your comfort and the stage of work you're in. Your birth partner, doula, or healthcare practitioner may support you in employing these approaches efficiently. Remember that every labour experience is unique, so discover the best tactics for you and your body.

Pelvic Floor Strengthening

Pelvic floor strengthening is vital for maintaining pelvic health, supporting your body throughout pregnancy, and preparing for delivery and childbirth. The pelvic floor muscles are crucial in managing bladder and bowel function, supporting the uterus, and aiding in the beginning. Here are some excellent strategies to improve your pelvic floor muscles:

Kegel Exercises

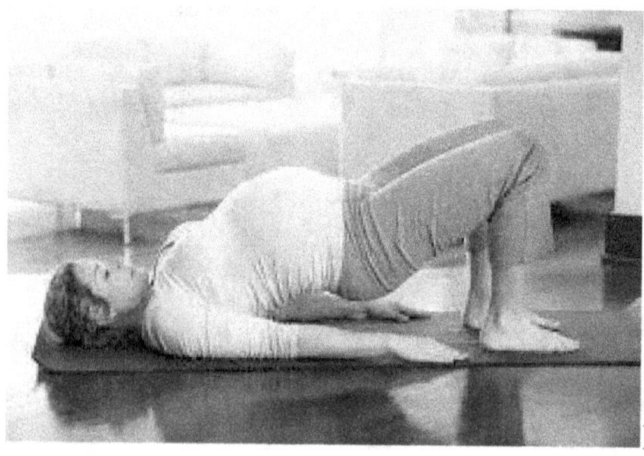

Kegel exercises are an excellent approach to preparing for labour and delivery, as they help strengthen the pelvic floor muscles that play a critical role throughout pregnancy, childbirth, and postpartum recovery. Strengthening these muscles may help greater bladder control, pelvic support, and general comfort. Here's how to practice Kegel exercises throughout the childbirth preparation period:

1. **Identify the Pelvic Floor Muscles:**
   - Before you start, find your pelvic floor muscles. You may accomplish this by thinking you're attempting to halt the flow of pee or avoid passing gas. The muscles you employ for these activities are called your pelvic floor muscles.

2. **Practice Proper Form:**
   - Sit, stand, or lay down comfortably. You can perform Kegels in any position.
   - Relax your thighs, buttocks, and abdominal muscles. Focus only on the pelvic floor.

3. **Engage and Lift:**
   - Contract your pelvic floor muscles as though you're attempting to raise them higher into your pelvis.
   - Hold the contraction for a count of 3 to 5 seconds initially.

4. **Relax and Release.**
   - Gently loosen the muscles and allow them to relax.

5. **Repeat:**
   - Start with ten repetitions at a time.
   - Gradually increase the time of each contraction as you feel more comfortable, aiming for 10-second contractions.

6. **Breathe:**
   - Breathe regularly during the activity. Avoid holding your breath.

7. **Consistency:**
   - Aim to complete Kegel exercises every day.
   - Incorporate them into your routine, such as completing them while brushing your teeth, sitting at your workplace, or watching TV.

Benefits of Kegel Exercises for Labor Preparation:

- **Pelvic Support:** Strengthening your pelvic floor may support the uterus and other organs.
- **Improved Blood Flow:** Strong pelvic floor muscles help promote circulation in the pelvic area.
- **Labour Preparation:** Engaging the pelvic floor muscles will help you become more aware of these muscles, which can be advantageous during delivery.
- **Postpartum Recovery:** Strong pelvic floor muscles may benefit in postpartum recovery, aiding with bladder control and healing.

Elevator Exercise

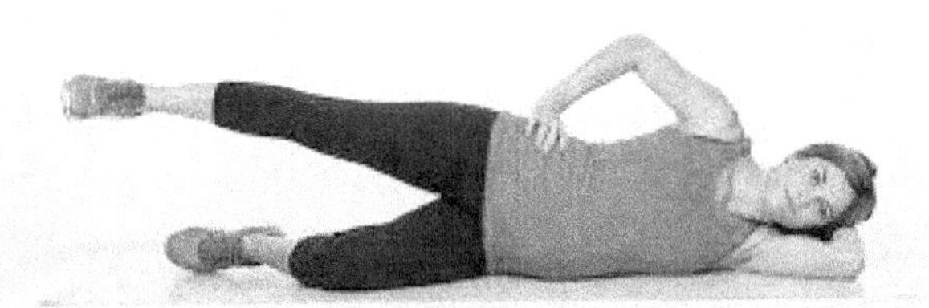

The Elevator Exercise is a version of Kegel exercises that focuses on varying degrees of activation in the pelvic floor muscles. This exercise might be especially effective during the labour preparation phase to strengthen and increase awareness of the pelvic floor muscles, which play a critical role throughout pregnancy, delivery, and postpartum recovery. Here's how to practice the Elevator Exercise:

Elevator Exercise for Labor Preparation:

1. **Find a Comfortable Position:**

   - Sit or lay down in a comfortable posture. You may execute this exercise in any pose that helps you to relax and concentrate.

2. **Identify the Pelvic Floor Muscles:**
   - Before you start, get comfortable with the feeling of activating your pelvic floor muscles. Imagine halting the passage of pee or avoiding passing gas to stimulate these muscles.

3. **Imagine an Elevator:**
   - Visualize your pelvic floor muscles as an elevator with several levels: the bottom floor, the first floor, the second floor, and so on.

4. **Start at the Ground Floor:**
   - Begin by gradually activating your pelvic floor muscles as though you're raising the elevator from the bottom level to the first story.

5. **Pause and Breathe:**
   - Hold the contraction at the first level for a few seconds, and remember to continue breathing properly.

6. **Continue Elevating:**
   - Slowly lift the "elevator" to the second level, then stop again and hold.

7. **Gradually Progress:**
   - Continue ascending and halting at each level, gradually going through the various levels.

8. **Hold and Release:**
   - Once you've reached the top floor (if you want to picture more levels), maintain the contraction for a few seconds, then gradually relax the muscles.

9. **Reverse the Process:**
   - Slowly lower the elevator to each level, halting and holding at each floor.

10. Fully Release:

- Finally, release the pelvic floor muscles entirely and allow them to rest.

11. Repeat:

- Practice this exercise for a few rounds, progressively increasing the time of the holds as you grow more comfortable.

Benefits of the Elevator Exercise for Labor Preparation:

- **Awareness:** This exercise helps you better understand varied degrees of involvement in your pelvic floor muscles.
- **Strength:** Practicing controlled contractions at different intensities helps strengthen the pelvic floor muscles.
- **Labour Preparation:** The activity enables you to connect with your pelvic floor, which might be advantageous during delivery.

Bridge Pose with Pelvic Tilt

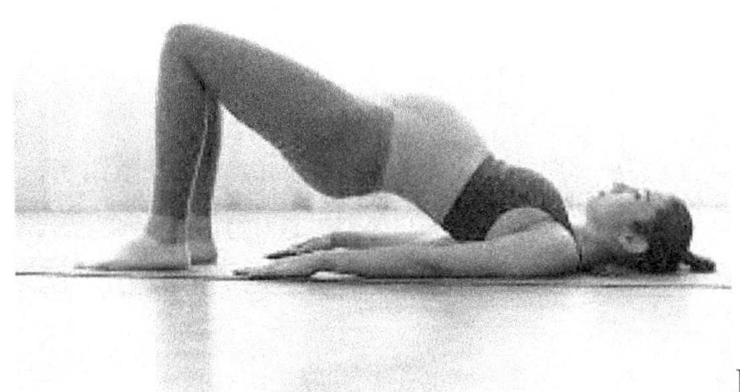

Bridge Pose with a Pelvic Tilt is a yoga position that combines the advantages of both Bridge Pose (Setu Bandhasana) and a pelvic tilt exercise. This combination may strengthen the pelvic floor muscles, activate the core, and enhance hip and spine flexibility. Practising this position throughout the labour preparation stage might improve pelvic stability and comfort. Here's how you execute Bridge Pose with a Pelvic Tilt:

Bridge Pose with Pelvic Tilt for Labor Preparation:

1. **Prepare Your Space:**

   - Find a comfortable and peaceful location to practice, such as a yoga mat or a cushioned surface.

2. **Lie Down:**
   - Lie on your back with your legs bent and feet flat on the floor, hip-width apart. Your arms should be lying beside your body, palms facing down.

3. **Pelvic Tilt:**
   - Inhale deeply, then as you exhale, contract your pelvic floor muscles and tilt your pelvis upward. Imagine squeezing your lower back against the floor while you tilt your pelvis.

4. **Lift Your Hips:**
   - Inhale again, and as you exhale, push onto your feet and raise your hips off the floor. Your spine should be rising one vertebra at a time.

5. **Support Your Hips:**
   - Slide your shoulders behind your back slightly, interlacing your fingers if you'd like. This offers support and stability to your hips.

6. **Pelvic Tuck:**
   - While maintaining the bridge posture, continue contracting your pelvic floor muscles and tuck your tailbone slightly under.

7. **Hold and Breathe:**
   - Hold the posture for a few breaths, concentrating on the engagement of your pelvic floor and the openness of your chest.

8. **Release and Lower:**
   - Exhale as you gradually release your hands and glide your spine down to the floor, one vertebra at a time.

9. **Rest in Supine Position:**
   - Take a minute to relax on your back with your knees bent and feet on the floor, experiencing the impact of the position.

Benefits of Bridge Pose with Pelvic Tilt for Labor Preparation:

- **Pelvic Floor Engagement:** The pelvic tilt activates and develops the pelvic floor muscles.
- **Core Activation:** The bridge posture engages the core muscles, improving overall stability.
- **Hip Flexibility:** The posture stretches and expands the hips, which may be helpful for pelvic comfort during pregnancy.

- **Spinal Mobility:** Rolling up and down through the spine increases spinal flexibility.

Squats with Pelvic Floor Engagement

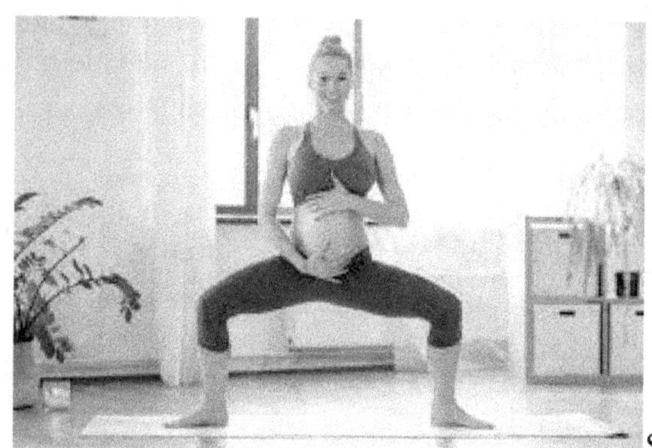

Squats with pelvic floor activation are an excellent workout to prepare for labour and delivery. Squats assist in strengthening the lower body muscles, increase flexibility, and activate the pelvic floor, which is necessary for sustaining the weight of the developing baby and aiding the delivery process. Here's how to execute squats with pelvic floor engagement throughout the labour preparation period:

Squats with Pelvic Floor Engagement for Labor Preparation:

1. **Find a Comfortable Stance:**
   - Stand with your feet slightly wider than hip-width apart. Toes may be slightly turned out.

2. **Engage the Pelvic Floor:**
   - Before you begin the squat, activate your pelvic floor muscles. Imagine raising and slightly tightening the muscles in your pelvic region.

3. **Initiate the Squat:**
   - Inhale as you bend your knees, dropping your hips down and back as if sitting in a chair.

4. **Keep Your Spine Aligned:**
   - As you squat down, keep a neutral spine. Avoid rounding your back or arching excessively.

5. **Engage Core Muscles:**
   - Keep your core engaged to support your lower back and stabilize your torso.

6. **Go as Far as Comfortable:**
   - Squat down as far as is comfortable for you. You don't need to go too low; strive for a comfortable range of motion.

7. **Push Through Your Heels:**
   - As you exhale, push through your heels and activate your glutes and quads to return to the beginning position.

8. **Continue Breathing:**
   - Breathe naturally during the action. Inhale as you sink into the squat, and exhale as you stand up.

9. **Repeat:**
   - Perform 10 to 15 repetitions, or as many as you feel comfortable doing.

- **Strengthens Lower Body:** Squats target muscles in the thighs, hips, and glutes, which may give more stability during birth.
- **Engages Pelvic Floor:** Engaging the pelvic floor during squats helps preserve pelvic floor health and prepares for delivery.
- **Promotes Flexibility:** Squats promote hip flexibility, which might be advantageous during labour and delivery.
- **Fosters alignment:** Proper squat form fosters a neutral spine and healthy posture.

Deep Belly Breathing with Pelvic Floor Engagement

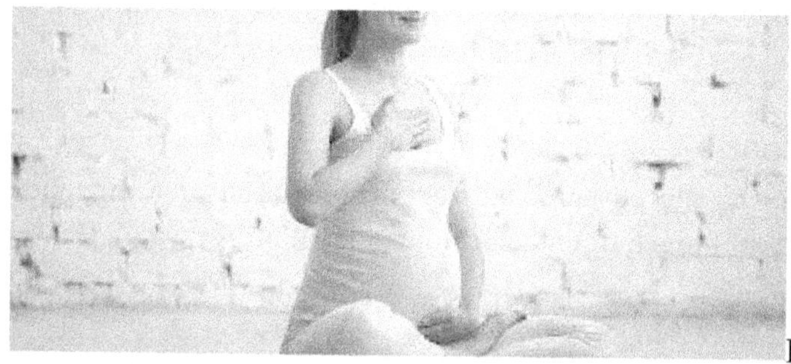

Deep belly breathing with pelvic floor involvement is beneficial throughout the childbirth preparation phase. It combines diaphragmatic breathing with stimulating the pelvic floor muscles, helping you connect with your breath, promote relaxation, and strengthen the pelvic floor in preparation for labour and deliveries. Here's how to practice deep belly breathing with pelvic floor engagement:

Deep Belly Breathing with Pelvic Floor Engagement for Labor Preparation:

1. **Find a Comfortable Position:**
   - Sit or lie down in a pleasant and peaceful location.

2. **Align Your Posture:**
   - Sit or lay with your spine straight and your shoulders relaxed.

3. **Place Your Hands:**
   - Place one hand on your chest and the other on your tummy.

4. **Inhale Through Your Nose:**
   - Take a steady and deep breath through your nose. Feel your tummy expand as you fill your lungs with air.

5. **Engage the Pelvic Floor:**
   - As you inhale, gently activate your pelvic floor muscles by thinking you're raising them upward.

6. **Exhale Slowly:**
   - Exhale gently and thoroughly through your lips, allowing your tummy to deflate naturally.

7. **Feel the Sensation:**
   - As you exhale, pay attention to the feeling of your pelvic floor muscles softly relaxing.

8. **Continue the Cycle:**
   - Inhale deeply, feeling your belly rise and your pelvic floor engage.
   - Exhale softly, allowing your tummy to sink and your pelvic floor to relax.

9. **Maintain a Rhythmic Breath:**
   - Continue this repetitive pattern of deep inhalations and gentle exhalations for numerous breath cycles.

Benefits of Deep Belly Breathing with Pelvic Floor Engagement for Labor Preparation:

- **Tension Reduction:** Deep breathing promotes relaxation and decreases tension and anxiety, helping you remain calm throughout birth.
- **Pelvic Floor Awareness:** Engaging the pelvic floor during breath training strengthens your awareness of these muscles.
- **Support for Labor:** The practice helps you gain control over your breath and pelvic floor muscles, which may be helpful during contractions.
- **Mind-Body Connection:** Deep breathing develops awareness and a deeper connection between your body and your breath.

Prenatal Yoga and Pilates

Prenatal yoga and Pilates are beautiful kinds of exercise for childbirth preparation. They provide a comprehensive approach incorporating physical postures, breathing methods, relaxation, and mindfulness, which may substantially aid you throughout pregnancy, labour, and delivery. Here's how prenatal yoga and Pilates might help you prepare for work:

Prenatal Yoga:

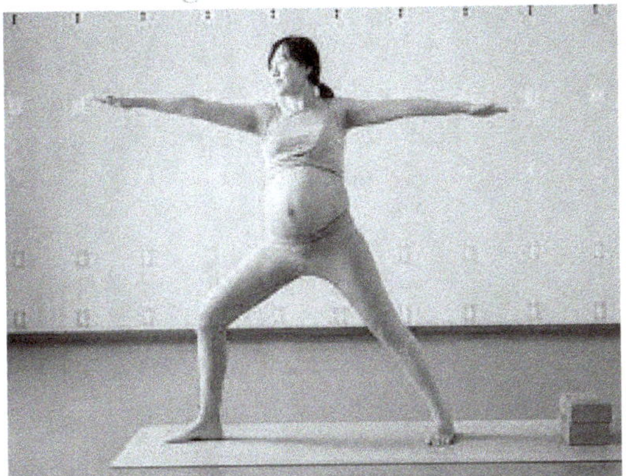

1. **Physical Strength and Flexibility:**
   - Prenatal yoga focuses on moderate stretches and postures that target multiple muscle groups, encouraging flexibility and strength.

2. **Pelvic Floor Awareness and Strengthening:**
   - Yoga typically integrates pelvic floor awareness and activation, helping you connect with these muscles and prepare them for delivery.

3. **Breathing Techniques:**
   - Prenatal yoga emphasizes deep and careful breathing, giving you the skills to be calm and centred throughout delivery.

4. **Relaxation and Stress Reduction:**
   - Yoga incorporates relaxation and meditation methods that help decrease stress, anxiety, and tension, establishing a good mentality for labour.

5. **Mind-Body Connection:**
   - Practising yoga develops attention and builds a deep connection between your body and mind.

6. **Adaptability and Modifications:**
   - Prenatal yoga sessions frequently give changes to meet your changing body and energy levels as your pregnancy advances.

Prenatal Pilates:

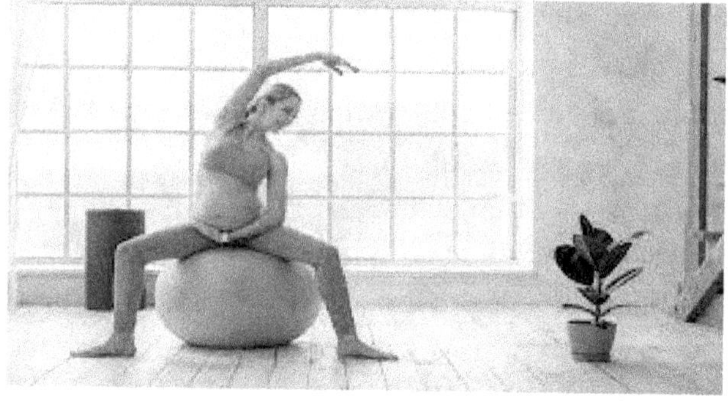

1. **Core Strengthening:**

   - Prenatal Pilates focuses on strengthening the core muscles, which may help your posture, stability, and comfort throughout pregnancy and birth

2. **Pelvic Stability:**
   - Pilates movements target the muscles that support the pelvis, boosting stability and minimizing pain.

3. **Breathing Coordination:**
   - Pilates emphasizes synchronized breathing with exercise, teaching you how to utilize your breath efficiently throughout birth.

4. **Alignment and Posture:**
   - Pilates may help improve your posture and alignment, minimizing pressure on your body as it adjusts to your shifting form.

5. **Low-Impact Conditioning:**
   - Prenatal Pilates delivers a low-impact workout that promotes cardiovascular fitness without placing unnecessary stress on your joints.

6. **Body Awareness:**
   - Pilates cultivates body awareness and fosters attentive movement, helping you become sensitive to your body's requirements.

Yoga Ball Exercises for Comfort

Using a yoga ball (also known as an exercise or birthing ball) during pregnancy may give comfort, relaxation, and support while your body experiences changes. Yoga ball movements may help ease back discomfort, improve posture, stimulate pelvic mobility, and even aid in preparing your body for delivery. Here are some yoga ball exercises for comfort during pregnancy:

Seated Bounces

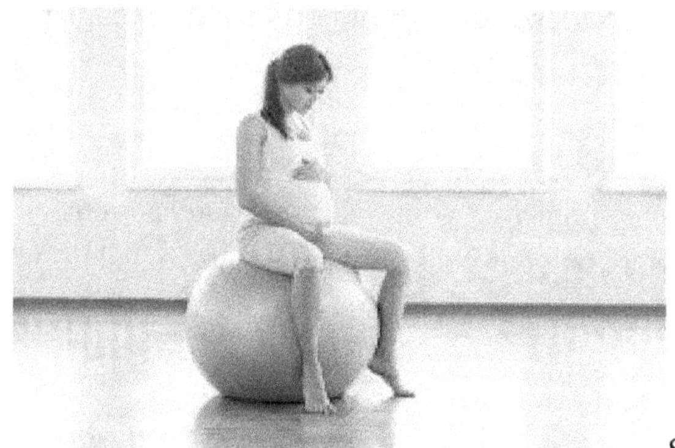

Seated bounces on a yoga ball might also be a good activity for labour preparation. The mild bouncing motion may assist in enhancing pelvic mobility, stimulate activation of the pelvic floor muscles, and give comfort during contractions. Listening to your body and checking with your healthcare practitioner before beginning any new fitness plan, particularly during pregnancy and delivery preparation, is vital.

Seated Bounces on a Yoga Ball for Labor Preparation:

1. **Choose the Right Size Ball:**
   - Make sure you're using a yoga ball that is the suitable size and height for you to comfortably sit on with your feet flat on the ground and your knees bent at a 90-degree angle.

2. **Find a Comfortable Space:**
   - Place the yoga ball on a solid surface where you may move securely and freely.

3. **Sit Comfortably:**
   - Sit on the yoga ball with your feet flat, hip-width apart, and your knees bent at a 90-degree angle.

4. **Engage Your Core:**
   - Sit up straight and activate your core muscles to maintain proper posture.

5. **Begin Bouncing Gently:**
   - Start slowly bouncing up and down on the yoga ball, allowing your pelvis to move with the action.

6. **Focus on Relaxation:**
   - As you bounce, concentrate on relaxing your lower back, hips, and pelvic region.
   - Allow the bouncing to create a sensation of comfort and release.

7. **Practice Breathing:**
   - Incorporate deep and rhythmic breathing while you bounce. Inhale as you rise slightly and exhale as you rest back into the ball.

8. **Pelvic Floor Engagement:**
   - As you bounce, intentionally activate your pelvic floor muscles with each bounce. Imagine raising and gradually tightening these muscles.

9. **Mindful Movement:**
   - Practice attentive movement and connect with the feelings in your body while you bounce.

10. **Listen to Your Body:**
    - Pay attention to how your body reacts if you experience pain; halt or adjust the action.

11. **Relaxation and Visualization:**
    - While bouncing, you may picture your pelvis expanding and relaxing, which might benefit birth preparation.

Benefits of Seated Bounces on a Yoga Ball for Labor Preparation:

- **Pelvic Mobility:** Moderate bouncing may increase mobility and flexibility in the pelvic region, which can be advantageous during birth.
- **Pelvic Floor Engagement:** Engaging the pelvic floor muscles may assist you in connecting with these muscles, boosting their reactivity during contractions.
- **Relaxation:** Regular movements and deep breathing may induce relaxation and alleviate stress.
- **Comfort during Contractions:** Seated bounces on a yoga ball give a pleasant method to move and sway during contractions.

Pelvic Circles

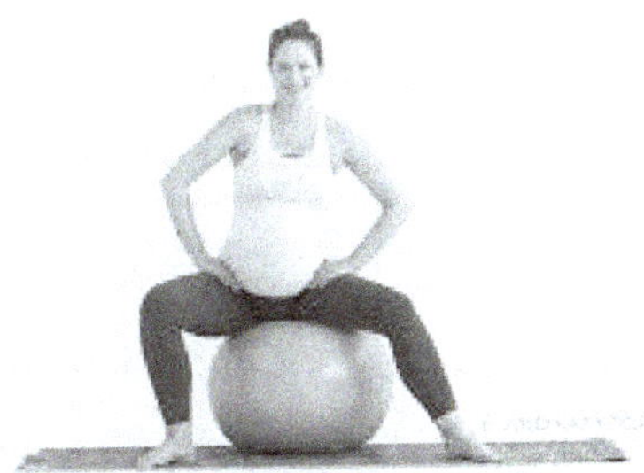

Pelvic circles are a gentle and effective exercise that enhances pelvic mobility, reduces stress in the hips and lower back, and prepares your body for delivery. This workout includes rotating your pelvis in circular patterns while sitting or standing. Here's how to conduct pelvic circles:

Pelvic Circles for Labor Preparation:

1. **Find a Comfortable Stance:**
   - Stand with your feet hip-width apart or sit on a firm surface like a chair or yoga ball.

2. **Engage Your Core:**
   - Whether standing or sitting, gently activate your core muscles to maintain your posture.

3. **Initiate the Movement:**
   - Imagine that your pelvis is the centre of a circle. Begin by softly leaning your pelvis forward (anterior tilt), then gradually

moving it to the right, turning it backwards (posterior tilt), moving to the left, and completing the circle.

4. **Complete the Circle:**
    - Continue the circular motion by tilting your pelvis to the left, pushing it forward, and returning to the beginning position.

5. **Reverse the Direction:**
    - After completing a few circles in one direction, reverse the movement. Begin with tilting your pelvis forward, then move to the left, then backwards, and complete the process by shifting to the right.

6. **Maintain a Gentle Pace:**
    - Perform the pelvic circles slowly and attentively, ensuring smooth and controlled movement.

7. **Breathe Naturally:**
    - Breathe normally during the activity. Inhale as you travel through one portion of the circle, and exhale as you complete the process.

8. **Focus on Relaxation:**
    - As you complete the pelvic circles, concentrate on relaxing the muscles in your hips, lower back, and pelvis.

9. **Perform Several Repetitions:**
    - Complete 5 to 10 pelvic circles in each direction, or as many as you feel comfortable performing.

- **Pelvic Mobility:** Pelvic circles increase the flexibility and mobility of the pelvic area.
- **Tension Relief:** The circular motion helps reduce tension and stiffness in the hips and lower back.
- **Labour Preparation:** Practicing pelvic circles helps increase awareness and control of pelvic motions, which can be advantageous during delivery.
- **Mind-Body Connection:** The practice fosters a mind-body connection as you listen to the feelings of your pelvis.

Hip Swings

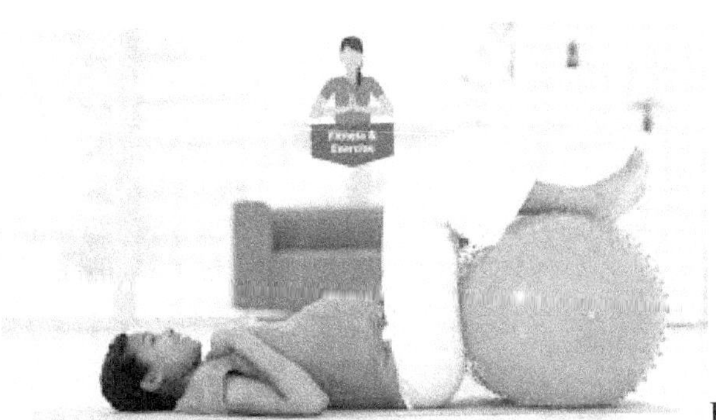

Hip swings are a mild and effective exercise that may assist in increasing pelvic mobility, reduce tension in the hips and lower back, and promote relaxation. This workout includes swinging your hips from side to side in a controlled manner. Hip swings might be very effective during pregnancy and birth preparation. Here's how to execute hip swings:

1. **Find a Comfortable Stance:**
   - Stand with your feet approximately hip-width apart. Make sure you're on a sturdy surface.

2. **Relax Your Body:**
   - Allow your body to relax, especially in your hips and lower back.

3. **Engage Your Core:**
   - Gently engage your core muscles to offer stability to your torso.

4. **Initiate the Swinging Motion:**
   - Shift your hips to the right, gently allowing your weight to migrate to that side.
   - As you do this, allow your left hip to travel outward to the left.

5. **Return to Center:**
   - Bring your hips back to the centre, keeping an upright stance.

6. **Swing to the Opposite Side:**
   - Now, shift your hips to the left, allowing your right hip to travel outward to the right.

7. **Continue the Swinging Motion:**
   - Alternate the side-to-side swinging action, allowing your hips to sway lightly.

8. **Keep a Gentle Pace:**
   - Perform the hip swings gently and attentively, ensuring the action is controlled.

9. **Breathe Naturally:**
   - Breathe normally during the activity. Inhale as you move to one side, and exhale as you return to the middle.

10. **Focus on Relaxation:**
    - As you practice hip swings, concentrate on releasing tension in your hips and lower back.

11. **Perform Several Repetitions:**
    - Complete 10 to 15 hip swings on each side or as many as feel comfortable for you.

Benefits of Hip Swings for Labor Preparation:

- **Pelvic Mobility:** Hip swings improve mobility and flexibility in the pelvic region, which might be advantageous during birth.
- **Tension Relief:** The side-to-side action helps alleviate tension and stiffness in the hips and lower back.
- **Mind-Body Connection:** The activity teaches you to tune into your body's motions and feelings.

Gentle Bounces with Deep Breaths

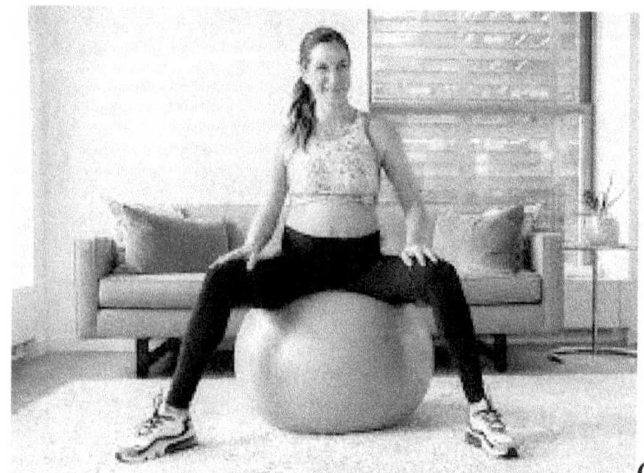

Gentle bounces with deep breaths are a peaceful and calming workout combining rhythmic movement and attentive breathing. This technique may help you release stress, improve relaxation, and connect with your breath as you prepare for labour. Here's how to conduct mild bounces with deep breaths:

Gentle Bounces with Deep Breaths for Labor Preparation:

1. **Choose a Comfortable Surface:**
   - Stand on a solid surface, such as a yoga mat or a carpet, in a calm, safe environment.

2. **Relax Your Body:**
   - Allow your body to relax, especially in your hips, shoulders, and neck.

3. **Stand with a Soft Bend in Your Knees:**
   - Stand with your feet hip-width apart and a gentle bend in your knees. This will give flexibility for the bouncing action.

4. **Engage Your Core:**
   - Gently activate your core muscles to maintain stability.

5. **Begin with Gentle Bounces:**
   - Start by slowly bouncing on the balls of your feet. Allow your heels to rise slightly off the ground with each bounce.

6. **Coordinate with Deep Breaths:**
   - As you bounce, match your breath with the action. Inhale as you rise slightly, and exhale as you settle back down.

7. **Maintain a Rhythmic Pattern:**
   - Create a moderate and regular pattern of bouncing and breathing that feels natural to you.

8. **Focus on Relaxation:**
   - As you bounce and breathe, concentrate on releasing tension in your body with each expiration.

9. **Visualize Relaxation:**
   - You may envision stress leaving your body as you exhale and serenity pouring in as you inhale.

10. **Continue for a Few Minutes:**
    - Aim to do this exercise for 3 to 5 minutes or longer if you find it pleasurable.

- **Tension Reduction:** The rhythmic bouncing and deep breathing may induce relaxation and relieve tension and anxiety.
- **Mindful Movement:** This practice increases awareness as you connect your breath with your movements.
- **Energizing:** The mild bouncing may assist in revitalizing your body and boost circulation.

CHAPTER NINE

Postpartum Yoga for Recovery and Rejuvenation

Postpartum yoga is a gentle and effective technique to promote your body's healing and renewal after delivery. It may help you restore strength, flexibility, and balance while fostering relaxation and mental well-being. Here's a guide to postpartum yoga for recovery:

1. Gentle Breath Awareness:

- Begin with a comfortable sitting posture. Close your eyes and concentrate on your breath.
- Inhale deeply through your nose and exhale slowly through your mouth. Feel the link between your breath and your body.

2. Pelvic Floor Exercises:

- Incorporate mild pelvic floor exercises to help restore strength and tone to these muscles.
- Inhale as you relax the pelvic floor, and exhale as you engage and elevate it softly.

3. Cat-Cow Stretch (Marjaryasana-Bitilasana):

- Move into a hands-and-knee posture.
- Inhale, arch your back and elevate your tailbone for a cow stance.
- Exhale, curve your spine and tuck your chin into the cat position.
- Repeat this flow slowly and carefully.

4. Child's Pose (Balasana):

- Sit back on your heels and drop your body between your thighs.
- Extend your arms forward or rest them beside your body.
- Allow your spine to extend, and concentrate on relaxation.

5. Bridge Pose (Setu Bandhasana) with Pelvic Tilts:

- Lie on your back with your legs bent and feet flat on the floor.
- Inhale to prepare, and as you exhale, raise your hips while contracting your glutes.
- Inhale at the top, then gently drop your hips down as you exhale.

6. Deep Belly Breathing:

- Sit or lay down comfortably and concentrate on deep, diaphragmatic breathing.
- Inhale deeply through your nose, allowing your abdomen to rise, and exhale slowly through your mouth.

7. Gentle Hip Openers:

- Practice mild hip-opening positions, such as the Butterfly Pose (Baddha Konasana) or Reclined Bound Angle Pose (Supta Baddha Konasana).

8. Seated Spinal Twists:

- Sit tall and slowly twist your body to one side, using your inhale to extend your spine and exhale to deepen the twist.

9. Legs-Up-the-Wall Pose (Viparita Karani):

- Lie on your back and put your legs up the wall.
- Relax and breathe deeply, enabling blood circulation to flow back to your heart.

10. Corpse Pose (Savasana):

- Lie down with arms at your sides, palms facing up.
- Close your eyes, relax, and concentrate on your breath.

Benefits of Postpartum Yoga for Recovery and Rejuvenation:

- **Muscle Recovery:** Gentle motions assist in muscle tone and flexibility recovery.
- **Stress Relief:** Mindful breathing and relaxation practices alleviate stress.
- **Emotional Balance:** Yoga fosters a feeling of tranquillity and connection with your body.

Pelvic Floor Rehabilitation: Yoga may assist in pelvic floor healing.

Increased Energy: Yoga helps decrease postpartum tiredness.

Remember that your postpartum body is unique, so practice at your speed. If you've had a cesarean delivery or other medical issues, see your healthcare provider before beginning a postpartum yoga practice. Start with shorter sessions and progressively increase the time as you feel comfortable. Most importantly, accept your body's demands and heed its messages throughout your postpartum journey.

CHAPTER TEN

Continuing Your Yoga Journey After Pregnancy

Transitioning Back to Regular Yoga Practice

Returning to your regular yoga practice after pregnancy involves care, patience, and attention. Your body has experienced enormous changes, so it's crucial to approach the shift gently and tailor your practice to your postpartum requirements. Here's a guide to assist you in negotiating this transition:

1. Consult Your Healthcare Provider:

- Before beginning any exercise, including yoga, visit your healthcare physician to confirm you're medically fit for more rigorous activity.

2. Start Slowly:
- Begin with mild postpartum yoga or modified variations of your typical positions.
- Focus on improving strength and flexibility while recognizing your body's present capabilities.

3. Listen to Your Body:
- Pay attention to how you feel during and after each session.
- If a position is uncomfortable or causes pain, alter or skip it.

4. Core and Pelvic Floor Strengthening:

- Prioritize core and pelvic floor workouts to improve stability and support.
- Gradually reintroduce positions that activate these regions, such as plank or boat pose.

5. Modify and Adapt:

- Use props like blocks, bolsters, and straps to assist your practice.
- Modify positions to accommodate any remaining soreness or stiffness.

6. Focus on Alignment:

- Emphasize good alignment to reduce strain and promote safety.
- Avoid deep backbends and severe twists initially.

7. Incorporate Breath Awareness:

- Practice deep breathing to reconnect with your breath and increase relaxation.
- Use your breath to direct your motions and maintain attention.

8. Be Patient and Kind to Yourself:

- Understand that your body may not return to its pre-pregnancy form quickly.
- Be patient with your growth and applaud every milestone.

9. Stay Hydrated and Nourished:

- Continue to focus on fluids and nutritional meals to help your recovery.

10. Get Plenty of Rest: - Adequate sleep and Rest are vital for postpartum recovery and general well-being.

11. Rebuild Stamina Gradually:
- Increase the time and intensity of your practice gradually.
- Respect your energy levels and avoid pushing yourself too much.

12. Connect with Your feelings:
- Recognize that feelings, such as joy, frustration, or vulnerability, are all part of the postpartum journey.
- -Allow your practice to be a place for emotional release and self-compassion.

13. Consider Postpartum-Specific Classes:
- Attend postpartum yoga courses created exclusively for mothers going back after childbirth. - These sessions provide a friendly setting and adaptations targeted to postpartum bodies.

13. Adapt for Breastfeeding:
- If breastfeeding, try yoga at times that don't conflict with your nursing schedule.

14. Stay Open to Change:
- Your practice may grow in unexpected ways afterwards. Embrace the changes with an open heart.

Transitioning back to regular yoga practice after pregnancy is a personal experience. It's a moment to recognize your body's power, perseverance, and the unique road it has gone. Approach your practice with self-care and a feeling of inquiry, and remember that every step you take is a step towards fostering your well-being.

Incorporating Baby into Your Practice

Incorporating your baby into your yoga practice may be a fantastic opportunity to connect, participate in mindful movement, and nourish your well-being while caring for your little one. Here are some innovative and safe ways to incorporate your infant into your yoga practice:

1. Baby-Wearing Yoga:
- Use a comfy and safe baby carrier to practice yoga with your baby close to your chest.
- Focus on gentle motions that assist your baby's safety and comfort.

2. Baby as a Prop:
- Use your baby as a mild weight or support in some positions.
- For example, cradle your infant in your arms during a chair pose or gently rest them on your legs during a reclining leg stretch.

3. Incorporate Baby's Movements:
- Engage in motions that naturally coincide with your baby's requirements, including swaying, rocking, or bouncing softly.

4. Partner Poses:

- Invite your infant to join you in partner poses, such as holding their hands during sitting forward folds or side stretches.

5. Baby-Enhanced Savasana:

- Lie down in savasana with your baby lying on your chest or abdomen.
- Embrace the connection and tranquillity as you both breathe together.

6. Playful Poses:

- Create a lively environment by including moderate motions your infant may appreciate, such as rolling side to side or elevating their legs.

7. Singing and Vocal Interaction:

- Infuse your practice with singing or humming, which helps relax both you and your baby.

8. Baby's Playtime:

- Practice yoga near your baby as they play on a mat or blanket.
- Engage with them via eye contact, smiles, and engagement.

9. Outdoor Yoga with Baby:

- Take your practice outside and spread a blanket for you and your baby.
- Connect with nature and let your baby explore their environment.

10. Guided Relaxation with Baby:

- Lie down with your baby near you and assist them through mild relaxation or meditation.

11. Baby-Led Practice: -

- Allow your baby's signals to direct your practice.
- You may incorporate more dynamic positions if they're content and alert. Concentrate on relaxing positions and gentle movements if they're tired or cranky.

12. Stay Safe and Attentive:

- Ensure your baby's safety by practising on a non-slip surface and avoiding positions that may jeopardize their comfort or well-being.

13. Enjoy the Moment:

- Remember that your practice with your infant is about connection and presence.
- Embrace the pleasure and spontaneity of practising together.

Incorporating your infant into your yoga practice may be a unique and enjoyable experience. However, always emphasize your baby's safety, comfort, and well-being. Your course may seem different today, and that's alright. The aim is to establish a loving and pleasurable atmosphere for you and your baby while you spend these precious moments on the mat.

Nurturing Self-Care as a New Mother

Nurturing self-care as a new mother is vital for your physical and emotional well-being. Taking care of yourself helps you and favourably improves your capacity to care for your kid. Here are some self-care techniques to consider:

1. Prioritize Rest:
- Sleep when your baby naps to optimize Rest.
- If feasible, ask for aid from your spouse, family, or friends so you can relax.

2. Practice Mindful Breathing:
- Take a few minutes during the day to practice deep, conscious breathing.
- This may help you handle stress and remain present.

3. Nourish Your Body:
- Choose nutrient-rich meals that offer energy and help healing.
- Stay hydrated by drinking lots of water.

4. Gentle Movement:
- Engage in mild postpartum yoga or stretching to alleviate stress and promote circulation.
- Listen to your body and avoid excessive workouts until you've recovered.

5. Connect with Support:

- Contact friends, relatives, or support groups to share your thoughts and experiences.
- Surround yourself with individuals who bring positive and understanding energy.

6. Accept Help:

- Allow people to help you with domestic work, cooking, and infant care.
- Accepting aid doesn't indicate you're incapable—it's a show of strength.

7. Set Realistic Expectations:

- Understand that it's common for things to alter after having a baby.
- Adjust your expectations and enjoy the new rhythm of your life.

8. Practice Mindfulness:

- Engage in mindfulness methods to remain present and build a feeling of tranquillity.
- This might help you manage stress and appreciate the tiny moments.

9. Express Your Feelings:

- Don't hesitate to discuss your excellent or challenging sentiments with a trusted friend or mental health professional.

10. Create Mini-Rituals:

- Find tiny moments to pamper yourself, such as having tea, bathing, or reading a book.

11.Stay Social:

- Stay connected with friends and participate in social activities that offer you delight.

12. Set Boundaries:

- It's normal to set boundaries and explain your demands to others, particularly regarding visits or social commitments.

13. Be Kind to Yourself:

- Avoid self-criticism and embrace self-compassion.
- Acknowledge that you're doing the best you can.

14. Get Fresh Air:

- Spend time outside to appreciate nature and get some sunshine.

15. Embrace Imperfection:

- Recognize that perfection isn't possible, and that's good.
- Embrace the glorious chaos of parenthood.

Remember that self-care is a constant activity, and it's not selfish—it's vital. Prioritizing your well-being helps you to be the most excellent version of yourself for your kid and your family. Celebrate every step you take to care for yourself as you traverse the fantastic adventure of parenting.